WHAT O1
BIRTH AN

"How extraordinary, and yet how simple, Marilyn's basic premise was: Birth, like conception, should be an intimate act between mother and father. No strangers necessary. Lovely stories, scientific evidence and Marilyn's wonderful commentary make this a must read book!"
- Laura Shanley, author of *Unassisted Childbirth*

"Marilyn Moran contacted me after reading something I had written in *The Compleat Mother* Magazine, to talk to me about intimate husband-wife birthing. She was intent on spreading the Good News about the way childbirth was designed to happen within a marriage. Her book was so eye-opening! After my husband and I experienced a private birth ourselves, I can only describe it as one of the most romantic things we have ever done. I am now also a 'Birth Evangelist,' sharing a better way to birth!"
-Sheila Stubbs, author of *Birthing the Easy Way*

"A classic! Must read for all couples planning to birth at home alone."
- Jenny Hatch, author of *A Lotus Birth*

"Game changer for me. First book I read on DIY birthing back in 1992."
- Penne Ard

"I have an original copy and it changed my life all those years ago."
- Wendy McNair

"Thought provoking....This book helped open my mind to the beautiful possibilities of birth and family life....I referred to it, reread it as I prepared for each of the births of my children (Five of my six were born at home). As I recently reread what I highlighted many years ago (my youngest child is 13) I remember the words that gave me not only

the confidence, but the desire to allow my husband to lovingly be the only attendant of our children's births. There is such a wealth of information contained in this book to help a couple prepare to lovingly birth their baby."
-Laura Hall

"If only we would begin relying on ourselves and our babies for direction. This Dyad (2) comes with very strong intuitive messages, if only noise around us could be MUTED so momma / baby would be able to communicate."
- Lynn Reed, Trust Birth Facilitator and Founder of Better Augusta Birth Experience (BABE)

"Moran's message is to let the 'love-gift,' the baby, come into the hands of the father. Anyone else present interferes with the bonding between the lovers - the birthing parents. This is the one book I would give to every pregnant couple to read - and all the birth attendants."
- Jeannine Parvati Baker, author

"*Birth and the Dialogue of Love* is a delightful collection of do-it-yourself accounts and convincing arguments. When the obstetrician is star, when the laboring woman looks at him with adoration after her child is born, when the new father is relegated to the minor role of hand-holding or brow-mopping, or when the midwife is seen as the one who 'made it all possible,' the three central figures lose their own importance, with devastating repercussions...*Birth and the Dialogue of Love* is one of the most important resources for committed couples approaching parenthood."
- *The Compleat Mother* Magazine.

"As one turns the pages with growing excitement, the positive reaction to Marilyn's theory grows ever stronger as she builds her case with judiciously selected facts from a wide variety of sources...What is the main point of *Birth and the Dialogue of Love*? Simply that wives and husbands

have so much to gain by sharing the birth experience by themselves at home. Marilyn does not categorically exclude the midwife or doctor, but she argues that the professional person should remain very much outside this crucial, critical moment in the couple's love relationship."
- Marion Sousa, author of *Childbirth at Home*

"The book is well worth reading and taking seriously, for its reminding factors about the archetypal images of marriage, intercourse and birthing can be of real benefit to attendants and couples alike…The primary value of the book, to my mind, is in consciousness raising so that couples and attendants realize the importance of birthing for the husband-wife relationship. How couples choose to manifest that should be their own choice."
- Rahima Baldwin, author of *Special Delivery*

"Marilyn Moran's *Birth and the Dialogue of Love* is ideal for couples wanting a homebirth, especially those choosing an unattended delivery to promote the father's active role in the birth process (which Moran maintains has been wrongly usurped by obstetricians)."
- *Mother Earth News*

"This book presents useful information on all aspects of homebirthing. Especially interesting are the sections on bonding and the importance of the senses and lactation, and on perineal massage and lovemaking techniques for easier, more harmonious and relaxed birthing. Her comparisons and contrasts of various methods of childbirth and their results are informative. Moran cannot detach birthing from sexuality; this may turn some readers off. But despite her attitude of 'knowing all the right answers,' her book presents a challenge to traditional thoughts on birthing and human development."
- Joan G. Easton

"Marilyn Moran, in her book *Birth and the Dialogue of Love*,

presents an enlightened message around the theme that childbirth is not only a natural, healthy experience but an important occasion for a husband and wife to grow in love for each other in a most profound expression of their love - a child being born."
- Lou Finocchario, MSW

"This is a book about love and childbirth. It is a book about giving and receiving. *Birth and the Dialogue of Love* sees birth as a 'love encounter.' It is filled with beautiful images of couple-shared childbirth through Marilyn Moran's inspiring visions, along with many quotes, poems and cartoons from various sources (shown in an impressive bibliography), and personal accounts of home births. In this book, birth is viewed as a natural, God given act of love in which husband and wife give and receive. It is seen as the ultimate climax of the act of love, with the father's hands the first to welcome the child into the world, with a focus on the psychological effects of birth on mother, father and child. These feelings are deeply explored and considered."
- Judy Grigsby

"Marilyn contends that the relationship between husband and wife would be greatly enriched if they shared the childbirth experience in the privacy of their home. To many readers, the very idea inspires questions like, 'Is it safe?' 'Is it possible?' 'Why would anyone want to do that?' and 'What do the health professionals and clergy have to say about it?' Mrs. Moran treats each question respectfully. She has certainly done her research. Thus, her book is not merely thought provoking; it is very informative."
- Bill Rose

"The gentle encouragement offered to home birth couples in *Birth and the Dialogue of Love* inspires courage. Many couples today are sensing the absurdity of allowing a masked stranger in white to position himself between a sterile-draped woman's naked legs for the purpose of

pulling out her baby. But a woman is fully capable of GIVING her birthing baby to waiting hands, and whose hands are more appropriate to RECEIVE her gift than those of her baby's loving father? Many couples, after reading this book, will come to this confident conclusion…Every pregnant couple will grow in confidence as they receive the comfort pouring from its innovative pages. For many, the encouragement will be like a breath of fresh air, just what they need to hear to experience the pinnacle of their love encounter of the best kind."
- Julie Butler

"For those of you who want to fully explore and experience the essence of human sexuality through conception and birthing; for those of you who want the new father to experience an active, not a passive role (holding the wife's hand, wiping her brow, or giving her a lollipop to suck), read *Birth and the Dialogue of Love*. Marilyn Moran feels that only the man who participated in the conception should be there to receive his wife's gift, their child."
- Jennifer Rodgers Gordon

"Moran presents these ideas in graceful and compassionate language, backing up many of her assertions with references to the growing body of literature on bonding and the psychological aspects of childbearing and sexuality. She presents her own version of 'do-it-yourself' homebirth, including suggestions for birth supplies and preparation and instructions to husbands for perineal massage. She concludes with a selection of nine birth stories which illustrate her ideas. Regardless of a couple's religious or political convictions, this book will help stimulate much-needed thought about the emotional aspects of birth for the mother and father."
- Janet Isaacs Ashford

Birth and the Dialogue of **Love**

By Marilyn A. Moran

Illustrated by Sandy Griffin

Terra Publishing

Tampa, FL

Copyright © 2019 Lynn M. Griesemer

Copyright © 1981 Marilyn A. Moran

All rights reserved. No part of this book may be reproduced in any form or by any means, except for the inclusion of brief quotations in a review, without permission in writing from the publisher.

Terra Publishing, Tampa, FL
ISBN: 978-0-9661066-6-4

Library of Congress Control Number: 2019912185

Cover design: Melanie Griesemer. www.melaniegriesemer.com
Cover Photo by Diego Ubiria

Permissions credits:

Margaret Gamper, R. N., and Midwest Parent-craft Center, for sketches from *Preparation for the Heir Minded*.

Dorothy Roberts and LaLeche League, Int., for "My Baby's Hand" which originally appeared in *LaLeche League News*, in about 1974.

DEDICATION

To my children and young lovers, everywhere.

Remember - "There are in the end three things that last: faith, hope, and love, and the greatest of these is LOVE."
1 Corinthians, 13:13

DISCLAIMER

This book is designed to provide information about the subject matter covered. It is sold with the understanding that the publisher and author are not engaged in rendering any psychological and medical advice or services. If expert assistance is desired or required, the services of a competent professional should be sought.

The purpose of this book is to share and encourage. The publisher and author shall have neither liability nor responsibility to any person or entity with respect to any loss or damage caused or alleged to be caused directly or indirectly by the information contained in this book.

TABLE OF CONTENTS

Foreword xv

Original Foreword xxiii

Introduction xxvii

Part One 1

1. THE TRUTH WILL MAKE YOU FREE 3

2. THE NESTING INSTINCT 17

3. BIRTH WITH DIGNITY 23

4. IF A CHILD COULD MAKE THE CHOICE 45

5. A TIME FOR RECEIVING 55

6. DOCTOR'S DILEMMA 69

Part Two 83

7. THE ENERGY OF LOVE 85

8. 21st CENTURY GOTHIC 89

9. MUSINGS OF A NON-SCIENTIST 95

10. COVENANT OF LOVE 103

11. TO FEMINISTS AND FRIENDS 107

12. PEACE IS A PAIR OF DOVES, UNFETTERED 111

Part Three 115

13. LOVE TALK 117

14. PREPARATIONS	121
15. FOR HUSBANDS ONLY	133
16. TEN USEFUL SUGGESTIONS FOR THE LOVING BIRTHING COUPLE	139
17. CARE OF MOTHER AND BABY	141
18. PERFECTION	145
Part Four	147
The Birth of Rebecca Lynn Crandall	149
The Birth of Luis Antonio Saavedra	161
The Birth of Hannah Smalltree	173
The Birth of Christopher Paul Dooney	179
Brad's Birthday	187
The Birth of Anna Marie Goodloe	199
The Birth of Jasmin Lutz	207
The Birth of Gabriel Arntsen	211
Shannon's Birth	215
Notes	221
Appendix	229
Suggested Reading List	231
Bibliography	233

About the Author 245

Two Poems 247

A note of appreciation 248

FOREWORD

Lynn Griesemer's Comments:

Marilyn Moran was born on April 11, 1928 and took her last breath on June 13, 1998. After the birth of her youngest son Patrick, almost 50 years ago, she became the first advocate for husband and wife, do-it-yourself homebirth.

Bob and I met Marilyn in December, 1997. One of her dreams was to organize a Husband and Wife Homebirth Conference, so we began planning the "First National Husband and Wife Homebirth Conference" for April, 1998. I can picture her gentle, affirming, passionate proclamation: "The husband gives his wife a love gift and nine months later, she gives the gift of a baby into his loving hands. She's present and accepting of his gift during coitus; he should participate and accept her gift during birth...At the moment of childbirth, when a woman is making her response to the genital gesture her man had initiated, no one should come between them then, not even briefly." She said, "It is imperative that couples abandon the doctors' quasi-pathological approach to birth...When an obstetrician steps in between the lovers at the moment of birth to catch the baby, the cyclic giving and receiving of significant genital gifts is shattered."

This is a challenging concept, given a culture that fears birth, conforms to a medical model, anticipates excruciating pain, and believes that a drugged childbirth experience is preferable. "Groundless fears and cultural taboos are the only obstacles holding her back from the goal nature intended that she achieve," says Marilyn.

Expectant parents are more often guided by culturally-induced fears rather than their desires and instincts. I believe that most men and women have a desire for a profound and satisfying birth experience. An obstacle to husband and wife birthing is the need to conform or belong. Marilyn describes a unique perspective on childbirth. Here, within these pages, she communicates what she passionately believes is the most desirable way to give birth.

Why aren't expectant mothers in touch with their instincts and desires for how they want to give birth? Are they afraid? Is the main goal annihilating the perceived pain? Do they want to by-pass birth altogether, instead, focusing on holding a new baby in their arms? Have they been swept up in expectations? Is it easier to conform rather than to do things differently from the norm?

When we abdicate our autonomy to medical personnel, we give up the power to embrace the present moment and natural flow of events. Institutional birthing comes with a high price: the possibility for a detached, disappointing, incomplete, disrespectful, or harmful birth experience.

Marilyn believed that birth was a dialogue, not a monologue. It is a dialogue between two lovers, and not intended to be a dialogue between a mother and an obstetrician. Marilyn and many others who've experienced this type of childbirth know that "childbirth is as much a part of the marital encounter as is coitus."

Giving birth in a romantic husband and wife encounter is a communication of love; anything less feels sterile and inauthentic. I can attest to the perfunctory, impersonal experience of childbirth in a hospital. I gave birth four times before I discovered that unassisted homebirth was one of the greatest joys on earth. Bob and I encourage young couples to consider unassisted homebirth. It was a pivotal point of our lives and still energizes us to this day, even though our two youngest children were born at home in 1996 and 2002!

The birth of a baby is an enormous life change for the baby and the parents. It's a defining moment for at least three people. Your life takes on a new dimension and you will remember the birth for the rest of your life. This one experience has the power to transform your entire being.

Times have changed since the 1970's and 1980's, where 50% of births involved anesthesia. Today, over 90% of hospital births include drugs. A higher percentage of first babies are born to well-educated and career-established women over 40 as well as unmarried women. More women are using medical procedures to conceive and bear children, which decreases the likelihood of a natural homebirth experience. In addition, single women are not likely to consider a couples' do-it-yourself homebirth either. And, the rise of a childfree by choice lifestyle continues to gain momentum. As I see it, husband and wife homebirth is not likely to be a consideration for many.

Marilyn published a quarterly newsletter, The New Nativity: A Newsletter for Do-it-yourself Homebirth Couples, which ran continuously for 25 years, under the additional names of Two Attune and The New Nativity II, and showcased over 300 birth stories. She's the author of *Happy Birth Days: Personal Accounts of Birth at Home the Intimate, Husband/Wife Way* (1986), and *Pleasurable Husband / Wife Childbirth: The Real Consummation of Married Love* (1997) in addition to *Birth and the Dialogue of Love* (1981).

This book will shatter your beliefs about childbirth. Originally published in 1981, *Birth and the Dialogue of Love* was out of print for a few decades. Because it's a classic birth book and truly one of a kind, we felt it would be important to offer a second edition. With a new cover design and a few typographical updates, we've kept the original content intact. Readers will find some of the medical information outdated, but the philosophies and birth stories timeless. The wisdom found within these pages is remarkable and can be life changing.

As you contemplate the concepts presented in this book, think about what it is you want for your birth. Is anything holding you back? Wouldn't you like to birth in a sensual, loving environment?

Lynn M. Griesemer
Author of *Unassisted Homebirth: An Act of Love*
www.unassistedhomebirth.com

Bob Griesemer's Comments:

Welcome to the re-published version of *Birth and the Dialogue of Love* by Marilyn Moran. This book completely changed my view of the act of giving birth and has a message that is sorely needed by a society that doesn't realize it needs it. My old view was the prevailing attitude that giving birth was a painful process my wife had to endure. It had to take place in a medical setting because of what could go wrong.

After reading this book, I changed that view into one that sees birth as the culmination of the conjugal act my wife and I engaged in 9 months prior. It's meant to be experienced by husband and wife in the intimacy of their own bedroom. If done this way, it can result in an experience that is so amazing I can only liken it to the psychologist Abraham Maslow's concept of a "Peak Experience." His description fit exactly what I experienced – a profound moment of love, understanding, happiness, or rapture, during which a person feels more whole, alive and self-sufficient.

Lynn and I struggled with whether or not we should publish this book given the current social climate related to marriage and family. The whole premise of this book is that marriage is a lifelong covenant between a man and a woman, the way God intended. Secular society used to agree with this, but it has been under attack for quite some time. The breakdown started with the implementation of the birth control pill which resulted in the movement to separate the act of giving birth from the conjugal act, as if the two were not related. Divorce laws were changed to "no-fault," where either spouse could file for divorce and the other couldn't do anything about it. Our society proceeded to legalize "same-sex marriage." If the conjugal act is rendered childless due to contraception and sterilization, then it follows that two men or two women can get married.

Let's add to this the advances in medicine. The medical establishment can do amazing things today that were not previously possible. I'm an example of that, having had a stent inserted into one of the major arteries leading from my heart, that was 80% blocked. I'm sure the stent saved me from a massive heart attack that could have ended my life.

Medical science can do some wonderful things to fix what is broken. The problem is the act of childbirth is not a "broken" process that needs to be fixed, but a part of women's nature that God designed. Women's bodies are made to give birth, which can be done without medical intervention. If done that way, it can be a peak experience the husband and wife will forever cherish.

So, here we are, with this book written by the late Marilyn Moran in 1981, with a message about the beauty of a married couple giving birth in the intimacy of their own home, in a current climate that doesn't value having babies. The birth rate is in decline in this country. Childbirth, it seems, has been relegated to an unfortunate process some women will go through, whether or not they are married. Where's the market for a message like Marilyn's that celebrates the love of husband and wife and the intimacy of the conjugal act in both its conception and its conclusion during birth?

I firmly believe there will come a day when the culture will be demanding information found in this book. Imagine that time, when we will come out of this social moral malaise, when intact marriages of husband and wife and family will once again be recognized as the foundation of a stable society and protected and encouraged.

This book is for you now if you are bucking those current trends in society and are married faithfully to a member of the opposite sex and the two of you are open to having children. You feel something is lacking in the medical model of childbirth that leaves you feeling that the husband has been left out of the process; deep down inside it doesn't seem right.

This book will open you up to the possibility that maybe, just maybe, that's not the way God intended when he designed us male and female, and that there is a better and more fulfilling way to bear children. That way is the husband's gift of his seed to his wife during the conjugal act and his wife lovingly returning that gift to him into his loving arms forty weeks later as a baby, truly the one flesh result of the union of husband and wife as the Book of Genesis tells us – "Therefore a man leaves his father and his mother and cleaves to his wife and they become one flesh." Gen. 2:24.

Let me end with a couple of quotes by Pope John Paul II, now Saint John Paul, who used that passage during his general audience on February 20, 1980 to explain in his *Theology of the Body* – "The body, and it alone, is capable of making visible what is invisible: the spiritual and the divine. It was created to transfer into the visible reality of the world the mystery hidden since time immemorial in God, and thus be a sign of it." On April 2, 1980, he said – "We are children of an age in which, owing to the development of various disciplines, this total vision of man may easily be rejected and replaced by multiple partial conceptions...Various cultural trends then take their place...Man then becomes more an object of determined techniques than the responsible subject of his own action."

Those are my favorite quotes from St. John Paul II's *Theology of the Body*, and I believe are directly applicable to the subject of this book. I'm sure Marilyn Moran saw that as she was writing this book at the same time. Do not become an object of determined medical techniques. Put into practice what Marilyn presents in this book and you will truly be the responsible subject of your own actions.

Robert E. (Bob) Griesemer, Jr.
October, 2019

ORIGINAL FOREWORD

This book is not just reading material. It is a vital experience opening perspectives most of us thought nonexistent. At the end you will feel sorry for those who have not experienced this work of Marilyn Moran, which explores human childbirth.

In less technologically developed countries it is common for women to deliver without the help of obstetricians. This has gone on for millennia. The American College of Obstetricians and Gynecologists was established comparatively recently.

Even at the University of Madrid, where I received my medical school training, a Spanish obstetrician with any self-respect would almost feel insulted if called to attend a low-risk mother in labor, more so if she had given birth before. These deliveries were customarily handled by midwives.

The United States has a higher neonatal mortality rate than many other countries. Hospital delivery is not the only answer to the problem. Many times the problem lies in the fact that the mother does give birth in a hospital, where doctors and nurses seem bound to administer medications which increase the rate of stillborn and blue babies.

Just a few years ago in this country it was common practice (and in some areas it probably remains so) to administer massive overmedication consisting of 100 to 200 mg. of Seconal (a barbituate) and 100 mg. of Demerol (a narcotic) and .4 mg. of Scopolamine (a drug which induces forgetfulness). This was repeated up to every two hours if the birthing mother but sighed loudly.

As a result the birthing mother was turned into a narcotized, belligerent, irrational, screaming creature who was trying to climb out of bed over the extra high bed railing. As soon as her cervix was fully dilated and the baby started to progress rapidly, the mother was shoved quickly to the delivery room where an episiotomy was performed and the baby delivered by forceps, as a general rule.

In contrast, in Madrid, with a midwife assisting at birth, perineal massage was the word of the day (in the 1950s) and perineal tears were few. The repair of those few tears was accomplished without the use of anesthesia. However, the joy of the occasion was such that even the stitching did not seem to bother the mothers much. I am not advocating suturing without anesthesia. I am just recalling what a moment of heightened emotion can accomplish better and with less side effects than medication.

My wife, Pat, who has given me five daughters and one son, has had spinal anesthesia for delivery several times. Once when she started delivering faster than the obstetrician would believe she could, she had an 'unplanned' natural childbirth. Her first remark about the experience was that it was a peculiar feeling, rather pleasurable, to feel her child come out during the actual birth.

Most of her deliveries were handled by the local intern or resident since the disbelieving OB would not come fast enough to the hospital. To top it off, the resident would wait for the private OB to come to the delivery room to look the "fait accompli" over and then the OB would come to the lonely I-wonder-what-is-happening fathers' waiting room and tell me, "You have a beautiful girl!" I would beam in joyful exultation and thank him effusively. A while later I would get to see my wife and then I would say to her simply, in a low voice, "Thanks." In this fashion we missed strengthening the bonds of our love as we could have. *She* should have been the recipient of my joy and thanks. *She* deserved them, not the OB. She should have seen my "virgin" (spontaneous) exultant rejoicing.

If she had witnessed my reaction at her birthing she would not have had silent fears about my not loving or caring about our first beautiful baby. I never used to hold our daughter. In Spain the old fashioned father would not handle babies much. Now that I have become more human and more "mothering," I enjoy cuddling and doing other things with my babies. They are never as lovable as when utterly dependent and small. When I do this, out of the corner of my eye I can see my wife smile and I realize that by loving my children our wife/husband love bond is strengthened. What a wasted opportunity for strengthening marital love it is not to share the birth of the fruit of our love! Just as we are the result of the creative love of God, so too our children are our love personified, the flesh and blood result of that which started initially as a platonic relationship.

This present work, by Marilyn Moran, is necessary if couples are to attain a higher stage in human development. How inhuman we have become is seen in persistent wars, injustices, and family disintegrations.

If humans have truly risen from the zoosphere (level of the animal), as Teilhard maintains, to the noosphere (level of knowledge), I dare say that there is another step fostered by the ideas presented here which can properly be called the amosphere. This lovesphere is the necessary prerequisite for the attainment of final fulfillment in Christo-genesis at the Omega point.

It is necessary for the grain of mustard to die in order for it to become a large plant where the birds of the air can make their nests. Out-dated scientific concepts, which turn out to be not only unnatural but also inhuman, must be discarded (at least their use as a routine mode of action). In a sense they must die so that the better, more loving, more human future can blossom. This will not occur without pain.

The uniqueness of the Christian message lies not in the love of neighbor, which is well set out in the Old Testament. The uniqueness of Christ lies in his revelation of the mystery of the cross. In a hidden way suffering has a redeeming significance. *Ad astra per aspera* - to the stars through difficulties. The way to the resurrection, to the rising to a totally new level of existence, lies only through the cross. There could have never been an Easter Sunday with its marvelous hyper-revelation and exulting super joy, without the sweat, tears, blood, suffering and death on the cross.

As a member of the medical profession I take my hat off to the insights presented in this book, and officially support their validity whole-heartedly. As a member of the human race I have nothing but thanks and admiration to give Marilyn Moran for her dedication and love which should have as their offspring a better future and more respect for life for generations yet to come.

J.C. Espinosa, M.D.
Cleveland, OH.

INTRODUCTION

Over the past five years there has been a noticeable increase in the number of homebirths that have taken place in this country. In a few rare instances the parents were able to convince a doctor to attend the birth. In other cases a midwife was located and persuaded to come and help, despite the restrictive laws of most states. More often than not, though, the couples chose to give birth without any assistance other than that of a friend or two who may or may not have attended a homebirth previously.

According to two studies the morbidity and mortality outcome of homebirths has been as good or better than that of hospital deliveries. Now midwives, both nurse and lay, are actively working to get prohibitive state laws changed so that they can assist a woman giving birth at home without fear of prosecution. They claim that men do not understand what it is to have a baby. Because of this, many midwives and feminists want the birth process taken out of the hands of the male-dominated medical profession and returned to the domain of women.

Although it is true that many women find a midwife more supportive and empathetic than a busy, male obstetrician, there is something extra special about giving birth at home with just one's husband sharing the mystical moment. Do-it-yourself homebirth mothers would not have it any other way.

The reason is that birth encompasses a relational aspect.

It is not just something that is happening to a woman. Rather it is something that is happening to a couple. As Sheila Kitzinger wrote, "It [birth] is part of a marriage and can enrich it or deprive it according to how the experience is lived through by both man and woman."

This book is an exploration of the interpersonal aspect of childbirth for husband and wife and its effect on their growth and development in two-in-oneness.

M. Moran

December 8, 1980
The Year of the Family

PART ONE

Changes in Due Time

MARILYN A. MORAN

1. THE TRUTH WILL MAKE YOU FREE

Whether one studies clouds in the morning sky, blossoms on a pumpkin plant, or the smiling face of a five year-old, one cannot help but notice the changes taking place. Clouds slip by, noiselessly shifting form and position, male blossoms close as female blossoms linger, inviting the attention of a stray, pollen-dusted bee, and the youngster may display a new tooth and a dozen freckles where previously there had been none. Change is a universal fact of life. There is no growth and development without it.

Socially, not all growth and development is docilely accepted however. There was resistance from the faithful when the Catholic Church abandoned its traditional fish on Friday law. Racial and sexual discrimination are illegal but many humans still suffer from both cultural holdovers. Education and understanding are required before the resistance dissolves allowing social changes to become the norm.

Beneficial innovations have been introduced regarding the experience of childbirth. They, too, have been met with resistance from some people, but with education and understanding that opposition will dissolve also.

Down through the ages women have generally given birth at home with the assistance of female relatives and friends. Except for herbal concoctions and prayers, there was little available to the laboring woman for the relief of her discomfort during the birth process. Suffering during childbirth, woman's penalty for transgression of the law of God in the Genesis story, seemed unavoidable.

Historically, surgical patients suffered greatly from intense pain, too. Although certain pain-killing drugs had been in use for thousands of years, they had only a small effect. It was not until 1846 that the first public demonstration of an operation under anesthesia was performed at Massachusetts General Hospital, in Boston, when a patient was administered ether.

Sir James Young Simpson, a Scottish doctor who was professor of midwifery at the University of Edinburgh, promptly introduced ether into his obstetric practice. The following year he published a paper on the advantages of chloroform over ether for both surgical operations and childbirth. Although the use of chloroform for the relief of pain in childbirth was violently opposed both on medical and on theological grounds, Simpson was undaunted. Finally, with the administration of chloroform to Queen Victoria at the birth of Prince Leopold in 1853, all opposition subsided.

The use of anesthesia during childbirth quickly became popular after it had been used by such a prominent person. If it was good enough for Queen Victoria, then it was just as good for commoners. During the century that followed its use was limited only by its availability.

For the convenience of the attending physician, the place for giving birth gradually shifted from the home to the hospital. There with several laboring women under one roof, the doctor could care for more mothers with less effort on his part.

Despite the enthusiasm of women for medicated childbirth, over the last few decades there has been a gradual shift away from the use of anesthesia during labor and birth. This trend is primarily due to the work of two men, Dr. Grantly Dick-Read of England and Dr. Fernand Lamaze of France.

Dr. Read at first practiced standard obstetrics, using

anesthesia. Once while assisting a woman in childbirth in a very poor section of London, and under very unfavorable conditions, he heard his patient say something which later caused him to reassess this approach to birth. He had wanted to give the young woman chloroform as the baby's head was crowning, but she declined his offer. Later when he asked why she had refused the chloroform she replied, "It didn't hurt. It wasn't meant to, was it, doctor?" [1]

In the following years, by carefully observing women in childbirth, Read deduced the fact that fear leads to tension and tension leads to pain which, not surprisingly, leads to more fear. By educating women about what is going on in their bodies during birth and by teaching them how to relax their muscles, Read was successful in converting the birth experience from a painful trauma to a joyous event for the mothers in his care.

In the meantime, Lamaze was developing a somewhat similar method of aiding the woman giving birth which subsequently eclipsed the work of Read. Lamaze adapted a method developed in Russia which was based upon the conditioning of reflexes as discovered by Pavlov.

The Lamaze method is termed psycho-prophylactic because it prevents pain from being registered in the brain by keeping the mind busy. Frequently an injured athlete will continue to play because in the excitement of the game he is unaware of his injury. Similarly, if the woman in childbirth is given an activity to distract her attention from her uterus, she will not perceive pain from that region of her body.

In the Lamaze method, controlled breathing is the activity which is used to inhibit the transmission of unwanted messages from the uterus and cervix to the brain. By accelerating her breathing as the contractions become stronger, the woman giving birth is able to tolerate them and not need anything other than this psychological anesthesia.

Both the Read and Lamaze methods permit the woman who is giving birth to gain control over her body. The former does this by having the woman focus inward toward what is happening inside her, the latter by having her look outward for distractions from what is happening inside her. Unlike Read, Lamaze places great importance upon the <u>monitrice</u>, or labor coach, to keep the mind of the laboring woman on her work.

A third person has made a significant contribution to the new childbirth. Sheila Kitzinger, a British anthropologist, childbirth educator, and mother of five children, has devised a method best described as psychosexual.

Kitzinger sees childbirth as one aspect of the total husband/wife relationship. Therefore, she assigns to the husband a role of great prominence. According to her,

> Parenthood...is part and parcel of the marriage and the love from the expression of which the baby owes its being. If this is so, our abilities as good mothers and fathers - and our failures too - cannot be viewed in isolation, apart from the sum total - <u>the interaction and fusing of personalities</u> [emphasis added] which makes up the marriage. This is one reason at least why birth is not merely a mechanical process of getting a baby born - nor should be even if it could be achieved. It is part of a marriage and can enrich it or deprive it according to how the experience is lived through by both man and woman.[2]

Because of the insights and efforts of Kitzinger and other current childbirth educators, as many as 50% of mothers who give birth at certain metropolitan hospitals in the United States today do so without anesthesia. Furthermore, most of these women have their husbands for support in the delivery room as their babies are being born.

It has been difficult for some people to accept this complete swing in the attitude of young couples from the traditional viewpoint that childbirth is a horrible ordeal to the new notion that birth is a positive experience to be shared fully by both man and wife. This new awareness concerning childbirth is really to be expected in view of the sexual revolution which has been perking away the past few decades. It has had an effect on the attitudes of even the most conservative people.

This is not to say that the young, denim-clad flower children are responsible for the current departure from traditional obstetrics. Back in 1959 Frances Freeh, author of the thought-provoking book about population decline, *The Great American Stork Market Crash*, gave birth to the first of three do-it-yourself homebirth babies, after having had five hospital deliveries. And it took Pat Carter only two hospital deliveries to make up her mind that there must be a better way. In 1957, when most of today-s homebirth mothers were themselves infants, she published *Come Gently, Sweet Lucina*, in which she described how and why she gave birth at home to her next seven babies.

Thoughtful, responsible women have been giving birth at home for many years, in preference to the hospital. Nevertheless, there is a cultural climate today which is conducive to the growth of new ideas concerning birth which have been quietly planted by others.

One such person who has contributed to the new awareness about birth is N. Kalichman, M.D. Back in 1951 he noted the similarity between a woman having a natural birth experience and a sexual experience and drew a graphic analogy between the two phenomena. In it he equated the descending baby with the male organ and wrote,

> ...as the climax is reached in both situations, the woman utters involuntary sounds and performs involuntary pelvic movements. With the expulsion of the child, as in reaching the climax of the orgasm, the woman suddenly relaxes, and there appears a calm ecstatic look on her face. The analogy applies as well at the post-delivery state. The woman's remarks are now directed to both the child and physician and are

usually tender and loving and are reminiscent of remarks following intercourse...As in intercourse the ideal may not be attained, and the expression of some of these various natural phenomena may be inhibited.[3]

In 1955 Niles Newton, PhD., enlarged upon the work of Kalichman. Using Dick-Read's observations of 516 women having a natural birth experience and the work of Kinsey, et al in describing phenomena accompanying a sexual experience, she drew an extended comparison between the two events and found a great resemblance between them. In regard to breathing, facial expression, uterine contractions, abdominal muscles, sensory perception and emotional response, coitus and childbirth, in Newton's words, are "strikingly similar."[4]

Without searching far, one may extend that list. In their book, *Human Sexual Response*, Masters and Johnson refer several times to the sex flush which appears on the neck and face late in the plateau phase of sexual response and "always identifies severe levels of sexual tension."[5] According to Jessica Dick-Read, widow of Grantly Dick-Read, "a flush also appears on the face of the woman giving birth when her cervix has dilated four centimeters, the appearance of which is a sure indication that labor is well in progress."[6]

Another phenomena that Masters and Johnson describe in detail is the carpopedal spasm, which is a grasping, clutching motion of the fingers accompanied by a curling of the toes. Like the sex flush, it appears in the late plateau phase of sexual excitement, and is another indicator of high levels of sexual tension.[7]

The carpopedal spasm also occurs during childbirth. In one of her earlier books Kitzinger said that if the woman giving birth "grips the bed, twists the sheet with her fingers or curls her toes," she is not relaxing properly.[8] Kitzinger did not use the term 'carpopedal spasm' but clearly that is it to which she is referring. In her more recent book,

Education and Counseling for Childbirth, she does use the term 'carpopedal spasm,' on page 185.[9]

Also, in a film of a homebirth which was shown at the Childbirth Speak-Out in Stamford, Conn., in June 1974, there was a segment in the film in which the camera had been focused on the woman's curling toes, i.e., the 'carpopedal spasm.'

That women experience uterine contractions during labor and birth is a well-known fact, needing no substantiation. Less well-known is the recurrent pattern of uterine muscle contractions during the orgasmic phase of female sexual excitement. Masters and Johnson even admit, "The contractile patterns are suggestive of those developed by the uterine musculature during the first stage of labor."[10]

There are other phenomena which occur in both coitus and childbirth, including hyperventilation, breast and nipple contour changes, as well as fluctuations in temperature and blood pressure. A final piece of evidence to be presented here showing the similarity between coitus and childbirth is a statement made by a young mother in describing her homebirth, at which time her husband 'caught' the baby. She wrote that as her labor came to an end, "with the next rush a baby squirted out of me into Aragyn's hands."[11]

Masters & Johnson drew a diagram showing the four phases of male sexual activity which basically looked like this:[12]

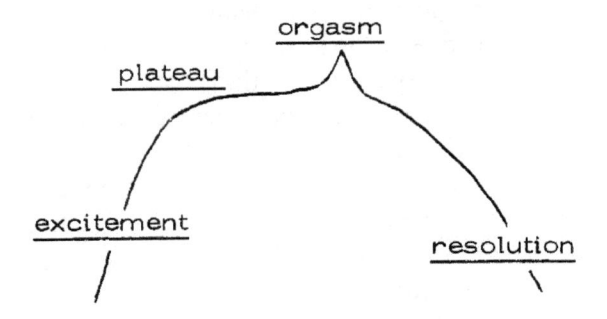

A line drawing showing the stages of pregnancy and birth makes an interesting comparison.

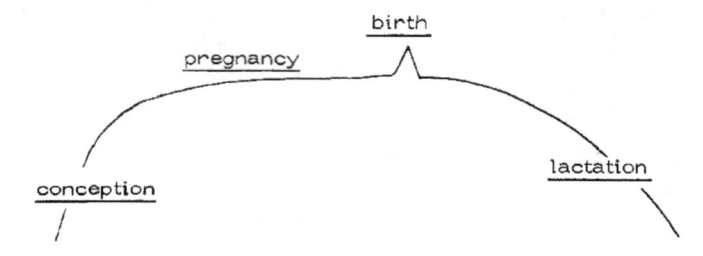

```
                    birth
         pregnancy   /\
              _____/  \_____
           /                 \
         /                     \  lactation
    conception                    \
       /                            \
```

The same general configuration can be seen in both the male sexual response cycle and the experience of childbirth, the ultimate orgasm for a woman. A man's genital gift-giving takes nine minutes; a woman's takes nine months. Time is hardly of the essence.

In view of all the evidence demonstrating the similarity between orgasm and childbirth, one finds perplexing the statement of Leon Chertok, echoed by others, that "one should remember...the basic fact that, in women, there is no necessary association between orgasm and reproduction..."[13] On the contrary, an objective analysis discloses a strong association between the two. As a matter of fact, the word 'orgasm' comes from the Greek word orgasimos which means 'to grow ripe, to swell.' That description certainly fits the pregnant woman.

Robert Bradley, M.D., a Denver obstetrician, uses the term 'birth climax' in his book, *Husband-Coached Childbirth*. He says that as the baby is actually coming out it is an exciting, provocative feeling for the unmedicated woman. According to Bradley's observations, the sensations she feels are comparable to those experienced in reaching a full sexual orgasm with the man she loves.[14]

Some women react to these sensations by wrapping their arms around their husbands' necks, squealing with delight, and beaming with ecstasy. "I always feel like an intruder and outsider to an intimate relationship between man and wife," writes Bradley. "I would feel embarrassed if the husband weren't there."

When two experiences are consistently described in the same terms, as coitus and childbirth are, those two experiences must be identical. Man's eyes are for taking in visual images no more and no less than woman's. Man's hands are for grasping and caressing no more and no less than woman's. When it comes to a genital expression, if coitus is, ideally, a communication of love and a unifying force, then the experience of childbirth must also be a communication of love and an equally unifying force.

Margaret Mead found that many so-called 'primitive' people recognize the sexual aspects of childbirth and for this reason prohibit men from seeing it.[15] If this detail has escaped the notice of the medical men in our culture they must be forgiven. Until recently most obstetricians were accustomed to coming into the delivery room moments before the birth, to find the woman a medicated, immobilized mass of matter with torso and legs so heavily draped that it would take a clairvoyant to discover that this was a human being making a significant human gesture.

When, as a medical student, Dr. Walter Menninger first observed a woman giving birth he found it so unsettling he was reluctant to discuss it with his wife. Calling it an "unforgettable scene" he wrote, "In the well scrubbed, cold hospital delivery room, the woman was already on the table, her legs in stirrups under draped sterile sheets. Gowned and masked nurses and doctors moved around her. I wondered how any woman could tolerate such an experience. Unquestionably, childbirth can be one of the most exciting and remarkable experiences in life. Regrettably, it is not always so. Sometimes it is not so because of natural complications; sometimes it is not so because the obstetrical management of birth becomes dehumanized and mechanical."[16]

Andre Hellegers, M.D., an obstetrician and director of the Kennedy Institute for the Study of Reproduction and Bioethics, criticized the books on the mechanics of sex by Masters and Johnson, saying they "are written as though no human beings were attached to the reproductive organs."[17] No doubt the same statement could be made about the obstetrical texts on doctors' bookshelves, from which they learned and to which they turn in reference.

Obstetricians are so concerned with cervical dilations and the descent of the baby that they cannot see beyond the other end of the uterus. Their myopia is revealed in a statement by another obstetrician who wrote, regarding the drugs used by American doctors, "scopolamine...tends to help the patient forget the torturous episode when it is over."[18] That line appeared in *Pregnancy: The _Best State of the Union*, by Waldo Fielding, M.D. How pregnancy can be such a great state and naturally end in a 'torturous episode' is beyond comprehension. It is incongruous. For something to end in a torturous episode the period prior to it cannot be sublime. It too must be distressful. After the first trimester, the majority of women find pregnancy a happy time of life. Therefore, it does not follow that it ends up the way that Fielding says it does. If indeed birth is a torturous episode it is because it has been made so.

Another obstetrician, listing the remarkable advances of modern obstetrics wrote, "We can get a cardiac patient through her pregnancy, tuberculosis is no longer a problem, and if a woman is potentially suicidal we can lock her up for nine months."[19] This reference to locking up the pregnant woman for nine months, by Robert E. Hall, M.D., then assistant professor of Obstetrics and Gynecology, Columbia College of Physicians and Surgeons, underscores the massive ignorance of men regarding the experience of pregnancy and birth for a woman and of her husband's role during the whole event.

Pregnancy can be a rich, rewarding experience or a nightmare. The pregnant woman is a person who has been put in orbit but unlike the conventional space ship hers is without controls. They are in the hands of her husband. When a breakdown in rapport occurs, the result is utter turbulence. Needless to say, any anxious moment experienced by the pregnant woman is also stressful to her man.

At the moment of conception an exquisite psychobiological ecosystem is established between man and wife of such fine nature that as many as 65% of first-time fathers experience some pregnancy symptom such as morning sickness, loss of appetite, or sleeping difficulty. Many times this happens even before the wife knows she is pregnant. Husband and wife are, so to speak, operating on the same frequency, from which everyone else is excluded.

This mutually beneficial symbiosis comes full circle at the love encounter of birth, which, strange as it may seem, is not 'splash down' but the apogee of the flight, the high point for the husband as well as the wife if (and only if) it is experienced together. As one new father said, "When our child was born I was the first one to touch it. Time stopped and it was the most real moment in my life."

The argument is raised, of course, that most husbands want no part of the birth experience. This is not surprising in view of the negative statements made by obstetricians for so many years. An example is the claim by William J. Sweeney, M.D., that "obstetrics is really a surgical specialty."[20]

That is enough to scare any young husband. Furthermore, a pregnant friend in New York City was recently given an instruction sheet by her obstetrician which stated, "Labor and delivery...should be approached without fear and anxiety." Yet in the following paragraphs, on the same page, the word 'pain' was mentioned twelve times. And on the top of the page, in bold lettering, was "TAKE PILL ON WAY TO THE HOSPITAL." Presumably it was some sort of a tranquilizing agent which had been prescribed. Such a recommendation generates negative feelings in a woman regarding the pending event. The effect is similar for her husband.

The same obstetrician's approach to childbirth was further revealed by certain phraseology on the instruction sheet. Never once was reference made to the mother giving birth. Instead the doctor used the words, "when your baby is delivered." In concluding he expressed the hope that the instruction sheet helped the mother to have a better understanding of what to expect "as the termination of your pregnancy approaches." [sic]

This man may know a great deal about the control of a technically-managed delivery, but clearly he knows nothing about the real experience of giving birth. And it is the likes of him that have been shaping the attitude of men and women toward birth for the last fifty years or so.

The aversion of husbands to participating in the childbirth experience is further understandable in light of the long history of men's exclusion from the birth chamber. In most cultures only female relatives and friends were called upon to attend a woman giving birth. And the tales these women had for their men-folk were none too cheering. (It is very possible these same women were grim about coitus, too.)

Nevertheless, birth is a normal, womanly, physiological function. Women are not biologically incompetent. They have been pre-programmed by their Creator for this act and are highly capable of fulfilling their biological responsibility. It is important, however, that no stumbling blocks are placed in their way by those who are needlessly fearful or those overly concerned with the technical details of birth.

There is a parallel between the new trend in childbirth and the recent trend back to breastfeeding. For a whole generation or more women in this country were persuaded that they could not breastfeed their infants. They were led to believe by their doctors that either their milk supply was inadequate, their milk was too watery, or else that they were too nervous. The work of the LaLeche League has proven to women, and to the medical profession as well, that women are biologically capable of breastfeeding their babies if they are given sufficient encouragement plus a few 'dos and don'ts' gleaned not from the professionals but rather from those women who have themselves successfully nursed their babies.

The problems encountered by the formula

manufacturers, as well as their solutions, are of no concern to nursing mothers. Women have nothing to learn from scientists in order to succeed at "the womanly art of breastfeeding."

Similarly, women are able to give birth consciously and joyfully, despite what they have been led to believe, and their husbands have much to gain by fully sharing the experience with them. All that they need are encouragement and a few practical techniques learned from other couples who have done it.

The sharing of the birth experience with one's mate is a uniquely human experience. But changing a thoroughly ingrained thought pattern is difficult. Because humans are capable of love, capable of reflection, capable of putting the real or imagined needs of the other ahead of their own personal inclinations, change is possible, however, and is coming about.

Throughout the country, thousands of husbands are remaining with their wives as they give birth. These men are finding it to be the most memorable experience of their lives. No man who has impregnated his loved one can remain a passive spectator while she gives birth to his child. Husband and wife are inextricably involved in each other psychically as well as physically. As he had participated in his wife's pregnancy, a husband can also participate in her birth experience with every fiber of his being, if only given the chance.

"Marvelous" is the word husbands most frequently use when they describe what it is like being present at their child's birth. It is not unusual for a husband to actually cry at that crucial moment. This was described by one father, when he first caught a glimpse of his daughter "still wet from the womb and all blurry from the tears in my eyes."[21]

He bent to kiss his wife and "our wet cheeks slipped comfortably against each other." The account continues, "Only then was I aware of the overwhelming wave of emotion that had been building inside me...part joy, and part relief, and part gratitude, but mostly pride: Pride in my newborn daughter, and pride in my brave wife, and pride in myself for just being present at this most perfect and beautiful of dawns."

Shared childbirth is a highly moving experience for both husband and wife. In the past men and women were taught that birth was horrible, messy, and nothing a husband should witness. This 'Chicken Little' fallacy is dissipating as recognition is made of the dynamic significance pregnancy and childbirth have for a man and woman in love.

2. THE NESTING INSTINCT

"If you want to get a good feeling inside, try holding a baby that is about 30 seconds old," advises Pat Kilcoyne, a young Chicago father who had that experience. "Like me, I don't think you can put it in words. The only way one can really know it is to do it."

Chicago's famed Maternity Center crew was late in getting to the Kilcoyne home for the birth of the couple's sixth child. But, surprising as it may be, that fact did not disturb Pat. "What made it even better is that there were just my wife, the new baby, and me," Kilcoyne related, proudly.[1]

An appreciation for privacy was also expressed by Larry Moots who assisted his wife, Vicky, when she gave birth at home to their third child. Asked what it was like to be the only person attending his wife, Moots said emotionally, "I can't explain it - my own, is all I thought."[2]

When a father supports the head of his child as it starts to emerge from his wife's body and feels the shoulders and torso slither out into his waiting hands, he participates fully in the birth experience.

To allow the father to participate in the birth on an experiential level is the reason why more and more couples across the country are trying their hand at do-it-yourself homebirth and are finding it the ultimate human encounter. But that is not the only reason why expectant parents are rejecting the standard hospital delivery in favor of giving birth at home.

Many women do not like rushing away to a strange, seemingly hostile environment. They are happier and more relaxed in familiar surroundings. They feel that labor is shorter at home than it would have been in the hospital because of the comforting feeling their own 'nest' provides.

Tonya Brooks, founder of the Association for Childbirth at Home, Int'l., surveyed fifty-one mothers who had given birth at home. The average length of labor for these women was five and one-half hours.[3] This is considerably shorter than the average length of labor for mothers delivering in the hospital in this country.

Prolongation of labor is only one of the results which occur when disturbing elements are introduced in the birth process. Niles Newton did research with mice to determine what effects handling the parturient animal had on newborn outcome. She discovered that among those animals whose nesting behavior was disturbed during labor and delivery the birth process not only took more time, but there were also more stillborn pups. In addition there was a longer period between births of litter mates as compared to animals in the control group which were not disturbed.[4] In another study it was demonstrated that the retrieving behavior of the mother animal was poorly established if she had been upset during labor. She failed to bring back and encircle those pups that strayed from her side.

Humans have a nesting instinct, too. They customarily knit booties and little sweaters. They borrow cribs and baby scales and give a fresh coat of paint to an old chest of drawers so that their 'nest' will be ready for the little one's arrival.

Many mothers even wash windows and iron curtains on the morning of the day that their baby is born. It is not by chance that women in the early stages of labor scrub their messy ovens with a new-found gusto. It is all part of that nesting instinct which nature has provided for both humans and animals alike.

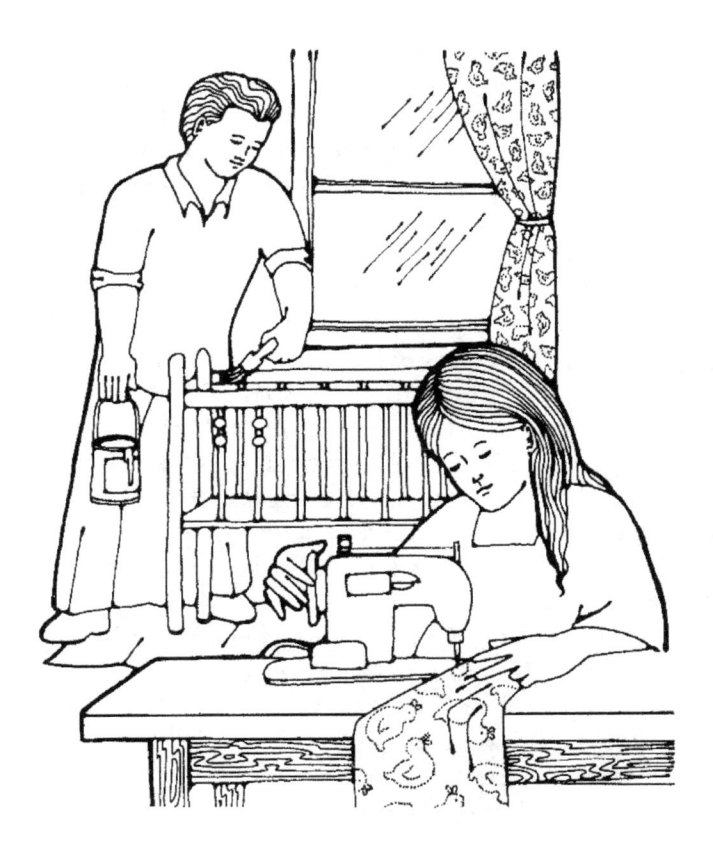

The mechanisms controlling the birth process are extremely delicate, subject to a variety of disturbances and more so among humans than among animals. The American culture requires mothers to give birth in a hospital. By custom mothers are removed from an environment in which they are content, and then subjected to handling by strangers with whom they are ill at ease in an environment that is strange and oftentimes frightening. Even the hospital odors carry the message to the laboring mother that this is not the ideal place for her to give birth. The hospital as an environment in which to give birth is so inappropriate that frequently the birth process slows down and even stops altogether.

Some mothers are giving birth at home because they

have found the hospital personnel to be indifferent, unsympathetic, and sometimes even crude in their remarks. Childbirth is the most important event physically and emotionally that a woman will face in her entire life. She deserves support and respect from her attendants at all times.

Other mothers are rejecting the hospital because the staff has preconceived notions which are antithetical to theirs. For example, Janet Darragh had Lamaze training in prepared childbirth when expecting her fourth child and was looking forward to a natural birth experience. However, without telling her beforehand, the doctor gave her a pudendal, a regional anesthetic, just before the baby was born. Janet was greatly upset by the doctor's action. "I felt it prevented me from feeling the baby slip out," she said. "That birth that I had looked forward to so much was disappointing to me."

In contrast, Carol Cronce, who gave birth at home, said she could feel the protrusion of the baby's nose as he was being born. She knew without looking that the baby was face-downward, so acutely aware was she of all the sensations of birth.

The immobilization imposed by the hospital gadgetry is what still other mothers resent. Many doctors feel it advisable to have an IV in place just in case it might be needed for the administration of medication. Others like to hook mother up to a fetal monitor. Both procedures limit a mother's ability to move about and find a comfortable position for giving birth.

At home mothers walk around, squat on their heels, and frequently assume a hands-and-knees position during labor and birth. These positions are more comfortable than the supine position. They also encourage the gradual dilation of the cervix, thus aiding in the birth process.

More than any other reason, though, mothers are staying home to give birth because they resent the forced separation of mother, father and baby. Birth is a bond-building event; the hospital routine has a devastating effect on the family's complex interpersonal relationships. Many couples see no salvation within the system despite some tokenism in recent years. The hospital stay is considered to be a period of psychic and physical deprivation for the mother, the baby, and the father as well.

Kay McMorris, after five hospital deliveries, gave birth at home to her next two children because "home seemed like the proper place to be born." After the first homebirth, Kay was about to cut the cord, when her husband indicated he wanted to do it.

Kay wrote, "I felt wonderful and he did, too. Dave was very proud of me and pleased with himself, and it was truly the best thing we have ever done together. He'll never forget, either. We often speak of it. It was really so simple and natural a thing. It seems unfortunate they can make such a mess of it culturally."

Neil Collins was also the only one assisting his wife when she gave birth at home to their second child. He expressed his feelings this way. "I came to see birth as a part of the love act between man and wife that does not require supervision any more than the act of conception."[5]

Cedar Koons echoed Collins' statement after she gave birth at home to her first baby. She said, "Stephen, my husband, caught the baby because we feel that birth is a deeply intimate act of love. It is something beyond conception. It is something that I think every woman should be able to share with someone in that bonding of love, experiencing and sharing with someone else the birth of her child. For me that someone was my husband."[6]

Not only is the husband-wife bond strengthened when father is included in the experience of birth, but the father-child bond is also strengthened. Mary Edwards had four medicated deliveries and then had a Lamaze baby, with her husband by her side. A few weeks later Mary overheard her husband calling the baby "my little girl." He had never spoken that way of the other children. Through no fault of his own, he apparently never felt as close to any of the other infants. Estrangement had been created by his exclusion from their births.

Fortunately, the fears and taboos surrounding childbirth are slowly disappearing. Husbands are being permitted to experience the birth of their children in a distinctively human manner, thanks to the providential yearnings which mothers become aware of as the time of birth approaches. In the past these yearnings were suppressed. But educated young women today are yielding to their deep-felt urges.

With minimum discomfort and maximum satisfaction women are giving birth at home. By responding to their nesting instincts mothers are achieving for themselves and their loved ones riches beyond measure. Mother, father, and baby in their own little nest -it is the ideal place for birth.

3. BIRTH WITH DIGNITY

A rose is a beautiful flower to see and it has a remarkably pleasant fragrance to enjoy. But, a rose if cut from the bush too soon will never unfold its petals and release its scent, and that which it was intended to do will forever remain undone.

Similarly, a married woman has a role to fulfill. Her calling is to bring peace to her spouse, and childbirth is an integral part of this assignment. At the moment of impregnation a man entrusts his most significant possession to his wife. For nine long months he anxiously awaits her response to his gesture. Unfortunately in our culture fears and taboos prevent her from responding appropriately to her man and achieving her goal of peacemaker. Her action is nipped in the bud and that which she is capable of doing remains forever unfulfilled.

Although women possess all the necessary faculties for giving birth, those in the culturally advanced countries have been led to believe that they are not able to do so. This is a myth, and unfortunately it is a myth that is believed as though it were gospel truth.

A certain government printing office pamphlet makes interesting reading on the subject. Emergency Childbirth was printed by the Civil Defense as a guide for assisting a woman giving birth in an air raid shelter. It states, "Let nature be your best helper. Childbirth is a very natural act...DO NOT HURRY - LET NATURE TAKE HER COURSE."[1]

Few people realize how natural an act childbirth really is. Most think birth is a crisis situation requiring technical management. This false notion can greatly complicate the task of the woman giving birth.

The Kansas City Times carried an article entitled "Baby Comes Into Cold World" which told about the hardship that one woman endured on the way to the hospital to give birth. The car in which she was riding was caught in snarled traffic because of a snow storm. In sub-zero temperatures she was forced to abandon the car and to walk, uphill, the last four blocks to the hospital.

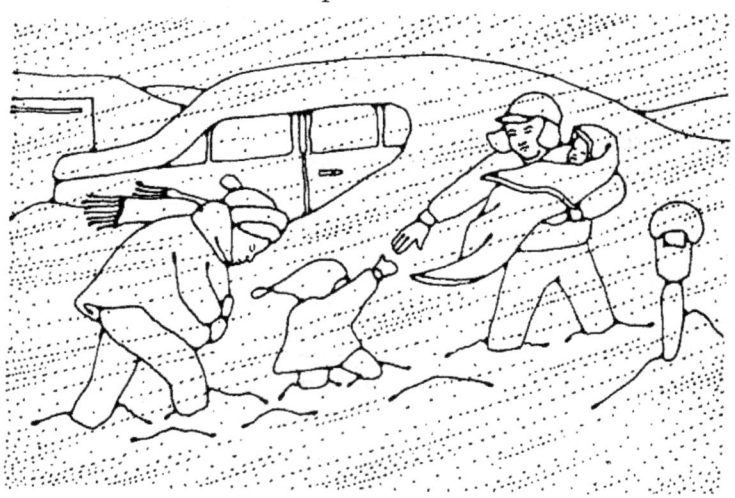

Her husband was carrying their seventeen month-old daughter while their six year-old, who was also with them, had to struggle along by herself. Fortunately, a passing motorist with snow tires stopped for the family about two blocks from the hospital and drove them the rest of the way. A half hour after arriving at the hospital the mother gave birth to a fine, seven-pound, two-ounce son.

What tension, discomfort, and trauma would have been avoided if this young woman only knew she could have stayed at home to give birth! According to the newspaper account, the father had driven recklessly in his attempt to reach the hospital before the birth of the child.

"I guess I did about everything," the father is quoted as saying. "I went the wrong way on a one-way street and drove on the wrong side of the street when traffic was backed up. Sometimes I was going 80 or 90."[2]

Clearly, the father was experiencing a crisis of his own. In addition, the little children were needlessly subjected to great discomfort during the mad dash to the hospital that cold and snowy morning.

The only good thing about the whole affair was that mother was on her feet and walking part of the time, thus gently aiding the dilation of her cervix. But she could have been doing that in her own kitchen as she made breakfast for the children, or while doing any one of a number of more pleasant occupations than taking that particular hospital trip.

There was no medically compelling reason why this mother had to go to the hospital to give birth. It is just that births customarily take place in the hospital in this country, that is all.

Too often the practices surrounding birth here have been developed with the doctor's convenience in mind, instead of the mother's well-being and ease. The best example of this is a practice that has been in use in America for the past forty years or more. Almost without exception, women have had to give birth flat on their backs with their feet up in stirrups to permit the doctor to follow the progress of the birth. This position is not the most desirable as it requires a tremendous amount of effort on the part of the mother to move the weight of the baby horizontally. Because of this handicap, labor is prolonged. Then the obstetrician must assist with forceps and/or an episiotomy, as well as with pain-relieving drugs.

All these interventions are avoided when mother gives birth at home. There mothers are not timid about assuming the squatting position, the universally-preferred one for giving birth. Otherwise, they sit, stand, or assume a hands-

and-knees position, whichever seems to be the most comfortable for mother at the time. In these positions gravity is working with them as they ease their babies out into this world.

Apparently the thought of squatting down to catch a baby is not to the liking of most obstetricians. At home the comfort of the mother is the primary concern, and the attendant's convenience is of minor consideration.

No one can tell the mother in which position she feels best. It is for her to discover. As in birth's counterpart, coitus, there is no right position; there are only preferred ones.

Another advantage to giving birth at home is that the mother can, and should, nurse her baby right away. Nursing is a comforting sensation to the child. It is nutritionally beneficial as well, for the first substance to be secreted from the mother's nipples is not true milk but rather colostrom, a fluid rich in antibodies.

Mother benefits from early lactation, too. The sensation of the infant's sucking triggers the release of a hormone, called oxytocin, into her blood stream. This hormone causes the mother's uterus to contract, which clamps shut the blood vessels at the site where the placenta had been implanted. Without this hormone, or a synthetic substitute, hemorrhage would likely occur.

A few years ago one mother lost considerable blood after delivering in the hospital. Although she was getting a transfusion and was receiving the hormone intravenously, her obstetrician became concerned. In an effort to prevent further blood loss he kneaded the mother's uterus internally and externally at the same time. Such a procedure is extremely uncomfortable.

Just prior to his ministrations, the mother said to the doctor, "How would it be if I nursed the baby? I understand this is very effective in getting the uterus to contract."

The doctor replied, "But, my dear, your milk won't come in for three days and we can't wait that long."

Whereupon he proceeded with his kneading technique.

Three years later this woman was again in the same room, same bed, having given birth to another daughter. Exactly four hours after the birth of the baby a nurse came trotting down the hall to the mother's room with the infant, so that mother could breastfeed the child.

Inquiring why this was so, when previously she had to wait twenty-four hours before being allowed to nurse, she was told, "In other cultures mothers nurse right away, and they don't have the trouble with hemorrhaging that we do. With your history of bleeding we don't want to take any chances, do we?" Mother nursed happily, and this time her uterus behaved as it should.

This mother had been one step ahead of her first doctor. Not only is nursing the baby a more gentle way to prevent hemorrhage, but it leaves no bruises.

Another questionable routine used in hospitals is forcing the expulsion of the placenta if it does not spontaneously deliver within a few minutes after the birth of the baby. Women who have given birth at home without medical assistance have discovered that by putting the baby to breast and waiting patiently the placenta will detach within thirty to ninety minutes with minimal loss of blood.

If the placenta is allowed to detach itself completely from the lining of the uterus, then there should be no excessive bleeding. Hemorrhaging occurs when the placenta is hastily yanked free.

Occasionally, when birth occurs at home without medical assistance, the placenta is not expelled for four or five hours. Sometimes the mother will go to sleep for a few hours and then expel it upon arising.

One doctor reports that in Vienna there is no concern about the placenta unless it is retained more than twelve hours. Unfortunately, the busy American doctor does not want to wait that long. He likes to have things all tidied up before he leaves the delivery room, and he has his own method of making the uterus cooperate.

The forceful expulsion of the placenta, in order to get

the mother out of the delivery room to make room for another delivery, or to permit the doctor to go on home, is a procedure prompted by the interests of the medical staff instead of the best interest of the mother. The whole situation is avoided when mother gives birth at home.

Incidentally, the previously mentioned Government Printing Office pamphlet, which had been prepared with the assistance of the American Medical Association, states, "Let the placenta (afterbirth) come naturally. Do not pull on the cord to hurry this process."[3]

The risks of homebirth have been greatly exaggerated. Also, mothers who have given birth at home are convinced that they and their babies are actually safer there than they would have been in the hospital.

John D. W. Hunter, M.D., assistant professor of Obstetrics and Gynaecology at McMaster University, in Canada, made an interesting observation which supports these women's convictions. After summarizing the risks of pregnancy he wrote,

> It is interesting that where pregnant women are left alone more, e.g., under the care of midwives or lay friends, the incidence of complications seems to be rather less than in those areas crawling with specialist obstetricians. This is food for thought, is it not?[4]

Lester Hazell, author of *Commonsense Childbirth*, and past-president of the International Childbirth Education Association, completed a study of 300 home births in the San Francisco Bay area. Her findings also support the wisdom of homebirth. About 10% of the babies in Hazell's study were delivered by doctors, and another 10% by lay midwives with little or no medical training but considerable experience with home deliveries. In the remaining 80% of the cases the mother was attended by only her husband or some friends. All these births occurred during the years 1969-1974.[5]

Among the 300 deliveries there was only one infant

death. The United States Demographic Yearbook for 1974 lists the following figures for infant mortality in the United States (per 1000 births):

1972: 18.5
1973: 17.7

For 300 births during either year, both of which occurred within the time-span of Hazell's study, the figures indicate a total of five infant deaths took place in the U.S. So, Hazell's homebirth population scored very well in comparison with the national picture, where the norm is delivery in the hospital.

In addition, in Hazell's group, there were no maternal deaths and only two cases of post-partum hemorrhage, both of which responded to remedial care at the hospital.

Granted, 300 is not a statistically significant number of cases upon which to draw any conclusions. However, for those who have been brought up to believe that one must go to the hospital to have a baby because a doctor is needed to do something at the moment of birth, Hazell's study reveals that it is not necessarily so.

Furthermore, some of the things which obstetricians routinely do in the hospital can have undesirable side effects. For instance both types of anesthesia administered in the hospital (general and conduction) "are associated with more blood loss after delivery, than occurs in an unanesthetized delivery, in which there is usually very little blood loss," wrote Constance Bean in *Methods of Childbirth*.[6] So, staying home to give birth automatically eliminates that cause of post-partum bleeding.

Another cause of excessive blood loss could be the anxiety created by separating mother and infant following birth. Emotional stress does have an effect on blood circulation. At home, with her newborn infant in bed with her, a mother is more apt to be calm and relaxed than she would be in the hospital with her baby in the nursery down the hall.

There are many reasons for the successful outcome of home births. Most of the women who choose to give birth at home are aware of the importance of good nutrition; they do try to eat intelligently, staying away from highly processed 'junk' foods and avoiding cigarettes, too.

The couples who give birth at home view childbirth as a normal, womanly, physiological function. Therefore, they approach childbirth calmly and confidently. Despite the evidence of the safety of homebirth for those who are well nourished, well read, and have received good pre-natal care, obstetricians still view homebirth with grave concern. The following story tells of a similar fearfulness on the part of a doctor, which didn't materialize.

A mother gave birth in the hospital to a little girl, who was promptly whisked away to the central nursery, as was the custom at this hospital. Therefore, the mother could not nurse the child for over twenty-four hours. Meanwhile, the doctor instructed the nurses to offer the baby water from a bottle. The baby refused to accept anything from a bottle, however. As the hospital stay progressed the doctor told the nurses to make her take it. Still, she adamantly refused.

Upon discharge the mother was told by the doctor (who incidentally was a woman), "I don't know what you are going to do if you ever lose your milk." Fourteen months later Claire Jean weaned her mother. The doctor's fears concerning the ability of the nursing couple to succeed were without foundation.

Similarly, the concerns of the medical profession regarding the ability of the prepared couple to bring the birth experience to a happy and successful outcome at home will also be without foundation in the vast majority of cases in which prenatal care reveals that birth will be normal.

There are several ways to demonstrate that homebirth is preferable to a hospital delivery. At home no harmful drugs are administered during labor. Mother and baby are not separated afterward. And a cause of sibling rivalry, mother's sudden departure and her later return with the new baby, is eliminated.

The most valuable but little-recognized evidence in support of birth at home, however, concerns the bond of love between husband and wife. There is a saying that "The past is prologue." What has gone before is the fore-runner of what is to come. Those same means used by the child in becoming bonded to his mother will later be used by him in becoming bonded to someone of the opposite sex. Therefore, by examining the manner in which a bond is spontaneously formed between mother and child one will perceive where couples err in the culturally constructed bond between husband and wife.

According to John Bowlby, M.D., the bond between mother and child is initially established when the baby smiles at mother and she smiles back. The "appropriate response" for the mother is to smile at the child. The infant's babbling and the mother's babbling back to the child further reinforces the all-important bond between them. If, however, the mother fails to respond appropriately, by mirroring the child's gesture, the child will withdraw and cease to smile and babble.[7]

Behavior initiated by one, <u>which elicits a like response from the other,</u> results in a strengthened bond between them. When mother does what the child does, she shows approval of the child and affirms his worth by becoming as the child is - a smiling, babbling creature.

Solidarity is demonstrated when one enters <u>fully</u> into the life of the other. Missionaries, Peace Corps workers, and diplomats have discovered this truth; they show unity with their host nation by adopting the ways of the people with whom they are visiting. To hold themselves aloof would be to perpetuate division and alienation and would be self-defeating.

The beneficial effect of openness to another was graphically illustrated in a film of Janet Adler, a dance therapist, interacting with an autistic three year-old girl. Amy was severely hampered in her ability to communicate. The therapist, by copying the postures and mannerisms of the child, was able to synchronize her movements with

Amy, thereby giving her someone with whom she could identify. At the end of the series of sessions Amy was gesturing when she wanted to be picked up, when she wanted to be swung around, and when she wanted to be held close, in marked contrast to her earlier behavior.[8] Only by entering into the life of the child was the therapist able to reinforce the self-worth of the child. By giving Amy good feelings about herself, Adler permitted her to slowly emerge from her isolated state.

<u>Son-Rise</u>, by Barry Neil Kaufman, tells of a similar emergence of the author's own son, Raun, from his state of autism. The toddler had a fascination for spinning plates and lids. So his parents decided to use this activity in an effort to make contact with him.

> We started to imitate him...for him, but also for us. Through our doing and repeating his behavior we hoped to find some relevant insight or understanding. We also believed that this was one of the few channels open to us through which we could let him know that we were with him. We wanted to use his cues as a basis of communicating....When Raun spun plates for hours at a time in a room, Suzi and I and whoever else was in the house would gather up plates and pans and spin beside him. Sometimes there would be as many as seven of us spinning with him, turning his isms into an acceptable, joyful and communal event. It was our way of being with him...of somehow illustrating to him that he was okay, that we loved him, that we cared and that we accepted him wherever he was.[9]

The efforts of the parents paid off and in time Raun started to smile at them, and to say words and to show an interest in his environment and the people in it.

The same bonding pattern which infants use in becoming bonded with their mothers (and which Adler and the Kaufmans also employed so effectively) can be seen in the developing boy/girl relationship. Boy smiles at girl. Girl smiles back. Boy speaks to girl. Girl speaks back. The handholding stage which follows is but an extension of this motif of behavior initiated by one eliciting a like response from the other with the result of a strengthened bond between them.

It is as though at each stage in the development of the affectional bond the young man voicelessly asks the question, "What does she think of me?" When the young lady makes the appropriate response, <u>mirroring his gesture</u>, he gets the message loud and clear, "I find you acceptable." If, however, she fails at any point to make the appropriate response, the developing bond is ruptured and the boy is free to enter into an affectional bond with someone else.

When the love relationship is finalized in marriage, and the young man bestows upon his beloved his most precious gift, his sperm, and conception results, again the appropriate response is for her to mirror his action and to personally give to him her most precious gift at the moment of childbirth. It is the only way to reinforce the bond between them. To turn to an outsider, an obstetrician, ruptures the developing bond between spouses and inflicts anguish upon one's husband not unlike that experienced by the infant who has been thwarted in his attempt to establish an affectional bond with his mother. For, to fail to affirm the worth of the other is to deny it. This is as true for the husband/wife dyad as it is for that of mother and child.

There is scientific support for the theory that childbirth is the moment for cementing the husband/wife bond. It is found in the study of critical periods in the development of social behavior. The general theory of critical periods for primary socialization, according to J.P. Scott, is that "the time when an organizational process is proceeding most rapidly constitutes a period when it (socialization) is most easily modified and this applies to organizational processes on any level."[10]

In other words, when there is a period of physical change and development, social interaction can be affected with lasting consequences. The author used weaning as an example of a physiological reorganization period. It involves a change in salt balance, fat intake, and general nutrition. According to Scott, weaning is a critical period for socialization because there is evidence that reproduction and other bodily functions may be affected when weaning takes place too early.

Probably the most well-known critical period is that for imprinting, a term coined by Konrad Lorenz, which in its generic sense implies the following: a) the development of a distinct preference; b) a preference that develops fairly quickly; c) a preference that, once formed, remains comparatively fixed.[11]

Shortly after hatching, for example, the young of many species of ground-nesting birds become attached to the first moving object to which they have been exposed, be it a bird of the same species, a wooden decoy, or even a human being. These 'imprinted' creatures stay close to the preferred object, emitting distress signals when out of sight of it, and contentment sounds when reunited.

Similar imprinting behavior has been observed in many mammalian species and the development of attachment behavior in human infants is comparable to that of sub-human mammals. The human infant develops a preference for one particular person during the first year of its life. Bowlby doubts the sensitive period starts before the infant is six weeks of age. By age six months he can usually track his mother both visually and aurally, and once he can crawl he will follow her, playing contentedly near her and showing distress when she leaves.

As the human infant develops physically at a slower pace than the young of other species, the exact points marking the beginning and end of this sensitive period for attachment with its physiological organization correlate is rather ill-defined. This is not so for the woman giving birth. There can be no doubt that she is undergoing an extensive physiological reorganization process as she changes from the pregnant to the non-pregnant state at the moment of childbirth. Her uterus will shrink, her breasts will become full, and even her ankles will grow slender once more, to cite but a few of the most obvious changes taking place within her body. The question might be asked, "At this critical period in her life what visual stimulus is she being offered as she gives birth in the hospital among strangers?" Whose smell is she being offered, whose touch, whose voice? The answer is obvious. The doctor's!

It is generally agreed that most women are in love with their obstetrician. Aljean Harmetz, writing in Today's Health, stated this quite boldly in recounting the birth of her third child.

> An hour late, my doctor comes, glib and beautiful...Can there be an ugly obstetrician? This lean, boyish-looking man with horn-rimmed glasses delivered both my sons. He - not my husband - is my partner in this intricate process. For a few days, emotionally, my child will belong to him. I will not say this to either man, but they will both know...The patients who do not fall in love with him hate his guts. None are indifferent.[12]

That quote comes, not from some women's glossy magazine, but rather from a publication of the American Medical Association!

Robert Bradley, M.D., also voiced the opinion that many women fall in love with their obstetricians.[13] He attributes the reason for this to the exclusion of their husbands from the birth experience. That is why he started to encourage them to come into the delivery room with their wives.

For the woman giving birth an obstetrician is a totally in-appropriate, though highly effective, 'imprinting' stimulus. The woman who develops an attachment for her doctor is no more able to act differently than Konrad Lorenz' goslings which waddle after him thinking he is their mother. Humans are subject to the same general laws of nature as are lesser creatures. The moment of birth is the magic moment for the woman to fixate upon a preferential someone. If the closest interacting person happens to be her obstetrician, then, for good or ill, she will become attached to him.

It goes without saying, that if she becomes attached to her doctor then the tie between her and her husband has become weakened. Once this happens there is no real marital union between them. Like a chain, the bond of love is only as strong as its weakest link.

Marshall Klaus, M.D., is a neonatologist at Case Western Reserve University who has conducted extensive research on bond formation between mother and child. His discoveries are relevant to the topic under discussion. According to Klaus if a mother is permitted to have her newborn infant naked in bed with her for one hour within the first three hours following birth, and is given five additional hours of contact with her baby each afternoon of the three days following delivery, her ability to 'mother' her infant is markedly improved. Those mothers, who were permitted early and extended contact with their infants, were given better scores in mothering thirty days later[14] and again one year later[15] than those mothers in the control group who were permitted only the limited contact with their infants that the traditional maternity hospital routine allows. (It consists of a glimpse of the baby shortly after birth, if mother is conscious, brief contact six to twelve hours later, and then when the baby is twenty-four hours old, visits of twenty to thirty minutes duration every four hours for feeding.)

Those mothers who had only limited contact with their infants displayed less interest and affection toward them later than those mothers who were permitted early and extended contact with their infants. For example, during a physical examination of their infant the mothers who had been permitted only limited contact were more apt to remain seated instead of standing by the infant and watching the proceedings. If the baby cried they generally made no attempt to soothe him. "It is surprising," wrote

Klaus, "with the multitude of factors that influence maternal behavior that just sixteen extra hours (of contact) in the first three days had an effect that persisted."[16]

Many animal mothers lose interest in their offspring when denied opportunity for body contact with them shortly after birth. Apparently the same is true for the human mother and infant. Similar deterioration in their ability to interact occurs if they are restrained from touch encounters during the critical bond-building period.

The behavior of each mother in the early and extended contact group was very interesting. When given her naked infant shortly after birth an orderly and predictable pattern of behavior was displayed. Starting "hesitantly with fingertip contact on the extremities, within four to five minutes (a mother under observation) began caressing the trunk with her palm, simultaneously showing progressively heightened excitement, which continued for several minutes. Her activity then often diminished, sometimes to such a degree that she fell asleep with the infant at her side."[17] (This behavior of the mother when united with her infant shortly after birth was considered comparable to the mutually beneficial licking and all-over nuzzling which many species of animal mothers engage in with their newborns.)

There must be something very significant about the progression from fingertip to palm contact. Among adults a handshake in which there is palm contact conveys considerably greater feelings of warmth and concern than that in which only the fingers are involved.

In comparing the behavior of the two groups of mothers,

Klaus and his co-workers found three measurements of interest and affection which they considered significant. They are the following:

1) <u>en face</u> – defined as the position of the mother's face held so that her eyes and those of the baby meet fully on the same vertical plane of

rotation. (see illustration)

2) touch – whether the mother's body was in contact with the infant's, and to what extent.

3) fondling – spontaneous actions of the mother not associated with feeding, such as kissing, hugging, stroking.

The researchers found marked differences in the behavior of the two groups of mothers in their interactions with their infants. En face, touch, and fondling were characteristic behaviors of the mothers who had been permitted early and extended contact with their infants but were missing in those mothers who were restricted to the traditional hospital routine.

One last point should be made here concerning observations of the importance of eye-to-eye contact of mother and child. Klaus found that both groups of mothers expressed strong interest in eye contact with their babies; he referred to the work of Robson,[18] who suggests that eye-to-eye contact is one of the innate releasers of maternal caretaking responses.

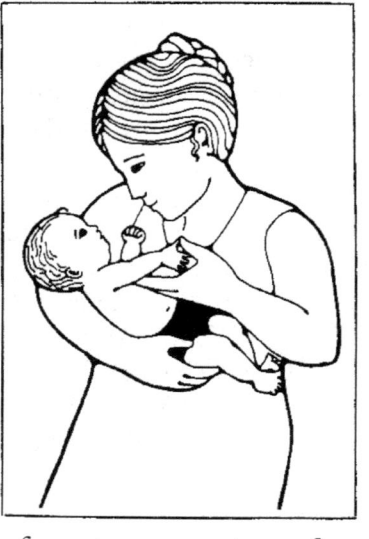

Because he is so tiny and helpless, the newborn infant must be irresistible to his mother so that she will give him sufficient care and attention to assure his survival. Klaus says the infant contributes to this bond formation, this lovemaking, with his eyes.

Normally at birth a baby has brilliant eyes and he can visually follow a person. Therefore, Klaus advises that silver nitrate not be put in the infant's eyes before mother and child have been reunited. Frequently this medication, which is used for the prevention of gonorrhea-caused blindness, causes the infant's eyelids to swell. When mother cannot see the baby's eyes, a delay occurs in the bonding process.

All these discoveries of Klaus and his co-workers about the mother-child bond are relevant to the bond between husband and wife, for their affectional ties are formed in the same manner and are just as easily disrupted. The same measurements of interest and affection which are applicable to the mother-child bond (en face, touch and fondling) are just as useful in assessing the strength of the bond between man and wife.

On the following page there are two pictures. One (Fig. A) illustrates the impediments to husband-wife bonding imposed by the hospital mode of delivery. In it there is neither <u>en face</u> positioning, touch, nor fondling between the marriage partners.

While it would be possible for the couple to make eye contact, the physical restraints imposed upon mother's body are a distraction. So are the medical attendants who would be giving instructions to the mother as she is about to deliver.

Touch by the husband is limited to lifting his wife's shoulders off the delivery table during a contraction to aid her in her efforts to expel the infant.

As for fondling, a husband can pat his wife's cheek, and stroke her hair, but little else.

Figure A

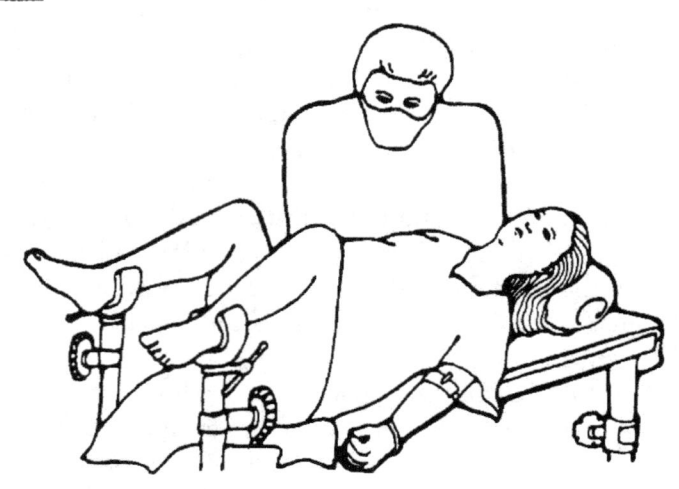

In contrast, birth at home as a love encounter is ideal for maximum interaction between man and wife. Figure B, of a couple giving birth at home, shows all three behaviors which are necessary for effective bond-building.

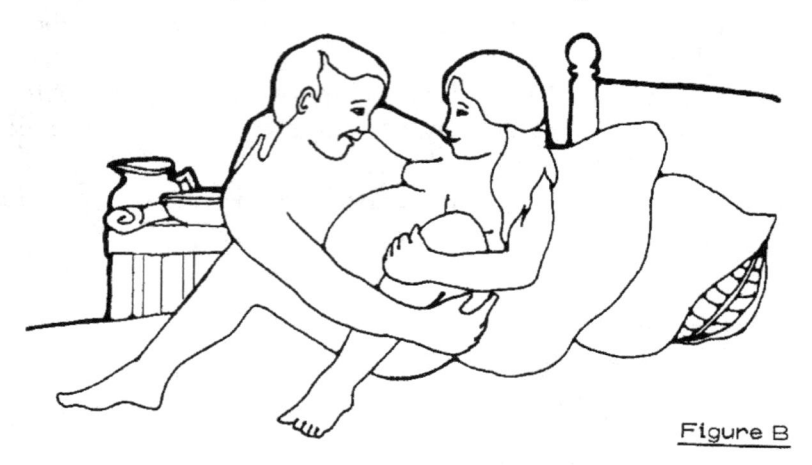

Figure B

Nothing and no one comes between husband and wife in the intimate, interpersonal experience of birth at home. Totally involved with each other, responding to each other, and oblivious to all else - it's possible at home and near-impossible in the hospital.

As for the important eye-to-eye contact in bonding, Eckhard H. Hess, in an article in *Scientific American*, makes some interesting statements about the significance of pupillary dilation. It is well known that the pupils of the eyes dilate or constrict in response to the amount of light present. But Hess discovered that they will also dilate or constrict in response to the amount of interest shown in the material viewed.

When a person shows interest in what is viewed pupillary dilation occurs, but a negative response causes the pupils to constrict. The ultimate negative response, not surprisingly, is to close one's eyes. Incidentally, pupillary changes occur in response to music and smell, which action indicates that the pupil is not only connected with the visual center of the brain, but also with other sensory centers.

One of the experiments conducted by Hess revealed the effect of a woman's eyes on a man. A series of pictures given to a group of twenty men included two of an attractive young lady, one of which was touched up to make the pupils of her eyes larger; the other was touched up so as to make her pupils smaller. A hidden camera recorded the men's reactions.

More than twice as many indicated a positive response to the picture of the young lady with large pupils than they did to the one with small pupils, although none of the men could tell why they found one girl prettier than the other.

According to Hess, "Clearly, large pupils are attractive to men, but the response to them - at least in our subjects - is apparently at a nonverbal level. One might hazard a guess that what is appealing about large pupils in a woman is that they imply extraordinary interest in the man she is with!"[19]

A woman's eyes are also dilating or constricting in response to the sensations she is experiencing while she is giving birth. If it is an exhilarating and ecstatic experience, her pupils should be saucerlike and, therefore, have an irresistible effect upon her man.

In a hospital delivery, however, bright lights are shone

down on the birthing couple. These lights cause the pupils of husband and wife to constrict. Furthermore, instead of gazing into each other's eyes in rapture, both shut them and grimace through the birth.

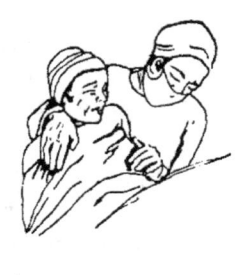

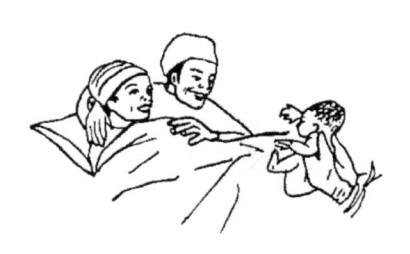

The above sketches appeared in *Preparation for the Heir Minded*, by Margaret Gamper, R.N.
Used with permission.

Granted, her man is by her side at the moment of birth. But without the assurance provided by his touch and with a negative response from his eyes, can a woman be certain of his interest and affection? And can he be certain of hers?

As Klaus said, regarding the mother-child relationship, "The affectional bonds of parents are very fragile and easily altered during those first days of life. One of the essentials of strong bonds of love is interchange. Parents and babies must be able to see and touch each other to make these bonds strong."[20]

Husband and wife, also, must see and touch each other if they are to succeed in forging an irrevocable union in marital love. In the typical hospital delivery the amount of opportunity for interaction between husband and wife is severely limited. Such restrictions cannot but have a damaging effect upon the quality of the marital bond.

One finds support for this assertion by again studying the work of Bowlby on the mother-child bond. According to him after the initial bond-formation period, if a baby has been adequately bonded with his mother there follows a phase in which the infant <u>resists</u> bond-formation with others. When approached by a stranger he fearfully retreats and clings to his mother.

Bowlby has seen some cases, however, in which this customary resistance to bond-formation was not displayed. In those cases the child had either been brought up in an institution or had experienced a series of foster homes; it had never been satisfactorily bonded to a preferential someone in the first place.

When an adequate bond has been formed, there follows resistance to bond-formation with others. But when the initial bond is inadequately formed this resistance is weak or lacking altogether.

The same is true for the husband-wife bond. Despite separation, if an adequate bond has been formed, resistance to bond formation with others will follow.

The nation's daily newspapers, with articles about marital infidelity and battered wives and statistics about the rising divorce rate, show how delicate and tenuous the marital bond is for many couples today. As Bowlby's work on bonding indicates such behaviors are only possible when the interpersonal bond has been inadequately formed in the first place.

Profound social and psychic costs are borne by couples whose babies are delivered in the hospital. With a doctor commandeering the event, a woman is prevented from responding appropriately to her husband in an effective manner.

Childbirth is not the time for a woman to get a baby but rather the time for her to give a baby to her beloved, bringing full circle that action which he had initiated nine months earlier. It is the moment for her to affirm his worth and to bring peace to her spouse. She is ideally endowed for consummating the marriage in such a singular manner. Groundless fears and cultural taboos are the only obstacles holding her back from the goal nature intended that she achieve.

4. IF A CHILD COULD MAKE THE CHOICE

"There is no more need to interfere with the course of normally progressing labor than there is to tamper with good digestion, normal respiration, and adequate circulation,"[1] wrote one prominent obstetrician. To interfere with the birth process can adversely affect the mother. The effect upon the baby can be just as distressing, if not more so.

Although some doctors interfere as little as possible, it has been customary in our culture to offer the laboring woman some pain-relieving medication. These drugs administered to the mother get through to the tiny infant within her and impair its ability to survive. The placenta, thought at one time to be a barrier, has turned out to be a bloody sieve. The following episode from *Woman's Doctor*, by William J. Sweeney, III, M.D., illustrates what can happen to the infant when its system is overloaded with medication that it cannot handle.

> By 9:45, Jean was having contractions every three minutes and feeling a lot of pain, even through the Demerol haze. My examination showed the cervix was eight centimeters dilated. I gave her a paracervical block, which is injected on both sides of the cervix, deadening the nerves in the immediate

area. It is an anesthesia I like a lot because the mother stays awake, and the baby isn't born groggy.[2]

The pages which followed contained a dramatic account of the drop in fetal heart rate, necessitating the use of forceps, and the birth of a "motionless baby...pallid, almost white." The doctor and the other attendants worked feverishly over the child, pumping oxygen into its lungs. Eventually the baby did respond and started to breathe, much to everyone's relief and joy. The doctor had no right to feel triumphant, however, for he may have contributed to the infant's distress by giving the mother demerol and the paracervical block.

Woman's Doctor was written in 1973.

One year earlier Doris Haire wrote *The Cultural Warping of Childbirth* and Constance Bean wrote *Methods of Childbirth*. Both authors criticized paracervical block anesthesia because of its tendency to cause the baby's heart to slow down.[3,4]

Furthermore, in 1970, obstetrician Watson A. Bowes, Jr., wrote, in *The Effects of Obstetrical Medication on Fetus and Infant*,

> Fetal bradycardia [abnormally slow heartbeat] following the injection of local anesthetic agents for paracervical block anesthesia has been noted for some time (Nyirjesy et al 1963)...Gordon (1968) published data showing that mepivacaine injected for paracervical anesthesia is rapidly absorbed into the maternal circulation and crosses the placenta to reach a peak concentration in the fetus about twenty minutes after administration. The concentrations of the drug were higher in those infants who had developed bradycardia than in those who had a normal fetal heart rate.[5]

It appears that the medication which Sweeney says, "I like a lot," turns out to be one that babies do not like at all.

The mother of this at-risk baby also received Demerol. It, too, has its undesirable effects upon the unborn child. According to Bowes' book on obstetrical medication, depression of respiration and decreased responsiveness of the newborn are two effects noted when this narcotic is given to the mother during labor.[6]

It is disheartening to realize how many obstetricians, unnecessarily, are still using anesthesia which can endanger the well-being of the infant. A drop in fetal heart rate means a diminished supply of oxygen to the infant's brain which causes neurological damage. At least 750,000 Americans are victims of cerebral palsy, a disability that stems from direct or indirect damage to the motor center of the brain before or during birth. Approximately 25,000 babies are born annually with the disability. In all probability it is the mismanagement of labor and delivery which is responsible for the children's difficulty. The excessive use of pain relieving medication seems to be the chief offender.

The position mother uses for labor and delivery can also affect the amount of blood and oxygen which reaches the infant's brain. This situation was discussed by Elliott H. McCleary in his book, *New Miracles of Childbirth*. The author interviewed Dr. Barry Schifrin, an obstetrician at Beth Israel Hospital, an affiliate of Harvard Medical School, who expounded on the marvel of the fetal heart monitor. This instrument measures the pulse and heart rate of the baby in utero and also the strength and frequency of the uterine contractions.

In the supine position, the one universally used in hospitals in this country, the heavy uterus may press on the mother's inferior vena cava and on the aorta, thus affecting the blood flow to her uterus. Any curtailment in the supply of blood to the uterus .means a curtailment in the supply of oxygen to the baby, which is so important for its brain. Monitoring reveals whether this has happened. Steps are then taken to correct the situation, generally by changing the mother's position from lying on her back to lying on her side. Without monitoring, the signs of asphyxiation can be missed.

Dr. Schifrin next referred to the work of Dr. William F. Windle, a researcher who temporarily asphyxiated monkeys immediately after birth. In so doing, he created both cerebral palsy and mental retardation in the monkeys. Asked if a great deal of the brain damage of infants could be prevented, Schifrin replied, "Much of it, because we're beginning to relate much of it to asphyxia - especially the asphyxia that develops during labor and delivery. We don't think that all the problems relate to this. Some are caused by disease, for instance, and poor nutrition. But asphyxia at birth is very important."[7]

Because of this connection between oxygen deprivation during delivery and brain damage, some obstetricians feel every birth should be guarded by an electrical monitor. A careful reading of Windle's work reveals no such necessity, however. In *Scientific American* Windle wrote,

> Spontaneous neurological deficits are practically unknown among rhesus monkeys born in their natural habitat or in colonies housed in laboratories. In this respect the monkeys differ from human beings.
>
> Most monkey births occur at night, as is the case with human beings. Labor is short: an hour or less. The female squats and drops the infant on the ground. During delivery most of the blood in the placenta passes to the infant and, as the uterus continues to contract after birth, the placenta is expelled...Human infants are born in much the same way in many parts of the world. The woman delivers, often unassisted, in the squatting position, and the infant, being below her, recovers most of the blood from the vessels of the placenta and the umbilical cord. . .In any delivery it is important to keep the umbilical cord intact until the placenta has been delivered. To clamp the cord

immediately is equivalent to subjecting the infant to a massive hemorrhage, because almost a fourth of the fetal blood is in the placental circuit at birth. Depriving the infant of that much blood can be a factor in exacerbating an incipient hypoxemia and can thus contribute to the danger of asphyxial brain damage.

In advanced countries, of course, the supine position of delivery is used to enable the attending physician or midwife to observe the birth conveniently and to assist if necessary. The squatting position, in addition to allowing the infant to receive the placental blood from above, has other advantages over the supine position. It avoids compression of the blood vessels supplying the placenta, which occurs in the supine patient when the gravid uterus tilts back against the pelvis.

The monkey experiments described in this article have taught us that birth asphyxia lasting long enough to make resuscitation necessary always damages the brain. This could be proved, however, only by histological examination. A great many human infants have to be resuscitated at birth. We assume that their brains too have been damaged. There is reason to believe that the number of human beings in the U.S with minimal brain damage due to asphyxia at birth is much larger than has been thought. Need this continue to be so? Perhaps it is time to re-examine current practices of childbirth with a view to avoiding conditions that give rise to asphyxia and brain damage.[8]

How carefully have Schifrin and his peers read Windle's work? Not very well, judging by the number of women who still give birth in this country in the undesirable supine position. It seems that Windle is saying, "Don't do it. Don't put the laboring woman on her back! Let her squat instead."

But the doctors select from Windle that which fits into their scheme, without creating too much disruption to their routine. Then they give the fetal monitor credit for saving the infants from brain damage, <u>after</u> the monitor has recorded the infants' distress.

Kermit E. Krantz, M.D., chairman of the Department of Obstetrics and Gynecology at the University of Kansas Medical Center, disturbed about the advent of home births, and implying that the hospital was the best place for birth, declared, "If a child could make the choice, he would desire every opportunity to be born healthy."[9] If a child could make the choice, he would not want his mother to be given anesthesia nor would he want her to lie on her back for his delivery. Both such dangers are avoided when birth takes place at home.

There are still other reasons why the hospital environment is not the ideal place in which to be born. As stated earlier, the most important criticism concerns the manner in which the hospital routine disrupts the bond-formation between the child and its mother.

It has been the custom of the hospital personnel to take the newborn infant from its mother the moment it was born. The infant was then kept in a central nursery where it was watched over and cared for by those supposedly more competent than the mother. She was given a few glimpses of her child and permitted to hold it briefly. At this meeting the baby was invariably bundled up in a receiving blanket. Even if the nurse did not specifically tell the mother not to unwrap the baby the mother usually hesitated to do so because she feared she would never be able to re-wrap the child in the exact manner. Mother's timidity about unwrapping her child delayed any finger-tip exploration of the infant's body, which should be followed by palm contact. It is just that type of contact that Klaus considers so important in mother's identification of and bonding with her infant. A few bold mothers would yield to their natural impulses, however, only to be later scolded for their actions.

A mother did not mind the scolding, though, nearly as much as she minded having a sleeping infant brought to her during the allocated time for nursing, only to have the baby continue sleeping, resisting all of her efforts to wake it. This can be very distressing, to be allowed only twenty minutes with your child and have her snooze the whole time, especially when you know she will be crying for you moments after being returned to the nursery.

In other little ways the hospital environment and routine disrupts the normal bonding sequence between mother and child. More than one mother has experienced dismay upon walking down the hall to the nursery only to find the curtain drawn across the nursery window, preventing her from getting even a glimpse of her little one.

The longer the delay is in getting acquainted and making eye contact the more seriously affected is the bond between mother and child. There is evidence that bonding between mother and child takes place in a critical period shortly after birth. How else can one explain the fact that although premature infants constitute only 6% of the baby population, between 25% and 40% of the battered children were 'preemies,' who had spent the early days of their life in incubators, where they had been denied their mother's gaze and touch. When the premature infants were finally united with their mothers weeks and sometimes months later, although they were physically fine they inherited a marred relationship. They were severely handicapped in their ability to cement a firm bond with their mothers at such a late date. Apparently the critical period for bonding is brief and cannot be recaptured once it has passed.

Despite inadequate bond formation with their premature infants, many conscientious mothers have been able to maintain a facade of tranquility. But for some mothers, when they are excessively fatigued or under pressure from other stresses, principally marital disharmony, their pretence cracks and their anguish reveals itself. Then innocent children become victims of the law of horizontal hostility. This law decrees that a person who happens to be in the wrong place at the wrong time becomes a surrogate victim for the one the distressed person really wants to injure.

Generally it is the spouse that the distressed mother really wants to wound, but it is the child of that spouse who receives the full effect of the pent-up anguish. This abuse can range all the way from broken bones and bruised flesh down to the lesser hurt of angry words and severe rebuke for minor infractions of the household rules. These can be just as damaging, psychically, over a prolonged period of time. The child who never succeeded in becoming adequately bonded to his mother is more vulnerable than any other.

But mothers are not the only ones suffering from deprivation in regard to contact with the newborn. Fathers, too, are in need of being bonded to their infants. Even more so than mothers they are shoved aside when birth takes place in the hospital.

The experience of Dr. T. Berry Brazelton, a prominent Boston pediatrician and author of several books on child development, will have a familiar ring for many fathers.

> At present, most hospital systems militate against a father's sharing the new baby with his wife. First the father is kept out of the delivery room. Next he's kept away from the baby by a glass wall. Then he must wait several days before he can assemble his family. By the time he takes his wife and 'her' baby home he finds that she has begun to cement her own relationship without him. Understandably, he feels left out and jealous.

> As an eager new father I was as surprised as most young fathers I talk to now that I really didn't feel as much emotion as I'd expected for the new baby, at least in the first eight weeks. In addition to a rather

remote interest in the infant, I felt estrangement from my clucking, involved wife.[10]

There is no reason why either father or baby must endure this eight-week estrangement. The child deserves and needs to feel his father's unconditional love from the very first. It should be loved simply for being. Such a love is possible if father and child are permitted to be in touch with each other during the all-important critical bonding period.

Recent studies indicate that the father's potential for establishing a life-long bond is much stronger at birth than later. Those fathers who are present during the birth experience become engrossed in their infants, being drawn to them like magnets.

An article in a regional newsletter of the International Childbirth Education Association illustrates the opportunity for cementing a bond of unconditional love between parent and child which is afforded in the immediate post-partum period. A physiotherapist had been in a hospital delivery room in the Netherlands observing how deliveries were conducted there when she saw a baby being born with a cleft palate. Immediately, she recalled the circumstances of a similar birth she had witnessed, in Canada. The Canadian doctor ordered the father from the delivery room, and had the mother 'put out' with general anesthetic. Later the mother's reaction to her infant was one of rejection.

Contrariwise, the doctor in the Netherlands, noticing the infant's disfigured mouth, placed a small gauze square over the lower half of the infant's face. He immediately held the child up for the parents to see, "Here is your son," he said. "He is beautiful. He has a cleft palate. First he will have a plate, and then in a few weeks, corrective surgery." The doctor then urged the parents to touch their child. The following day when the therapist and the doctor visited this couple, the parents were holding the infant and cuddling him. His face was not covered and during the visit the guests heard the mother proclaim, "He is beautiful!"[11] For the parent's growth and development into other-centered human beings, and for the most beneficial vibrations and sensations in which to enfold a newborn infant, there is no better place for giving birth than the parent's love-nest. There all are safe from the harmful effects of meddlesome interference. The little one will breathe in love, success, and self-worth through the pores of her skin. She will thrive-primed by the tones of loving voices, the touches of loving strokes, and the scent of parents totally dedicated to each other and to her. If a child could make the choice that is what she would ask for.

5. A TIME FOR RECEIVING

When Queen Victoria accepted chloroform for the birth of Prince Leopold, the trend was started for shifting birth from the home to the hospital. Laymen could not be entrusted with the responsibility of administering anesthesia. It was a saving of the doctor's time if all the women he was attending were under one roof and he did not have to travel from place to place. Then, as now, there was a shortage of doctors who had to be accommodated.

When the location for giving birth was shifted from home to hospital, not only did the mother welcome the change, but her husband also considered it one of the benefits of modern progress. Aware that mothers and infants sometimes died during childbirth and aware of his responsibility for her present condition, a husband felt great relief knowing his beloved wife was in the hands of the most competent person for her safe delivery and that of their baby. Professionals took over the management of childbirth, and man and wife yielded to their expertise.

Although a man can detach himself spatially from the birth of his child, he cannot detach himself emotionally. When a man impregnates his loved one, something vitally important to him goes out from himself. It is for this reason that frequently the husband of a pregnant woman experiences pregnancy symptoms.

Many times this occurs even before his wife is aware

that she is pregnant. The 'mind of the body' knows it, even though, consciously, he may not. From the moment of conception on, a husband is actually in an altered state of consciousness. He remains thusly until that moment nine months later when he personally discovers all is well and that which he had given away is recovered.

In our culture, however, a husband is denied the opportunity to participate in the birth experience in a significant manner. Generally, he has had no choice but to wait out the long hours in the Father's Room at the hospital until given the good news of his wife's safe delivery.

"It is an unwritten rule that nobody talks to the husband until the doctor officially brings the news. This is a privilege, for it is almost always an experience of pleasure and amusement," wrote Waldo L. Fielding, M,D.[1]

The long and stressful wait is not pleasant for the new father, however. The "Fathers Only" Journals of the Chicago Wesley Memorial Hospital reveal that the hours of waiting are anything but amusing. As one father wrote during the lonely vigil, "Becoming a father is tough on a guy."[2]

"Oh, God, be with Emma - she needs you right now even more than I do," conveys the anguish of one husband when separated from his wife at the moment of childbirth.

The uniqueness of the childbirth vigil is disclosed in, "My wife, Kate, is late as usual. She is never on time for any damn thing." If this man's wife were undergoing any other hospital treatment, such as an appendectomy, he would never experience irritation. His feelings would be only of sympathy and concern.

The husband of a woman giving birth is simultaneously going through a crisis of his own, and most people fail to recognize this. For the father-to-be in our culture childbirth is a time of frustration and agony. This is not fair.

The French obstetrician, Frederick Leboyer, maintains that babies should be born in a quiet, dimly-lit room to ease their transition from the uterus, where light is soft and sounds muffled to the noisy, daylit, atmospheric world. He decries the current treatment of the newborn. Babies have been penalized, says Leboyer,[3] because they are not able to verbally communicate their needs and preferences.

Husbands, too, have been penalized because of their inability to verbalize their needs regarding childbirth. In other cultures, many of which we would term 'primitive,' this penalizing has not occurred. In them it was recognized that childbirth was a tumultuous experience for a husband, and efforts were made to ease his discomfort.

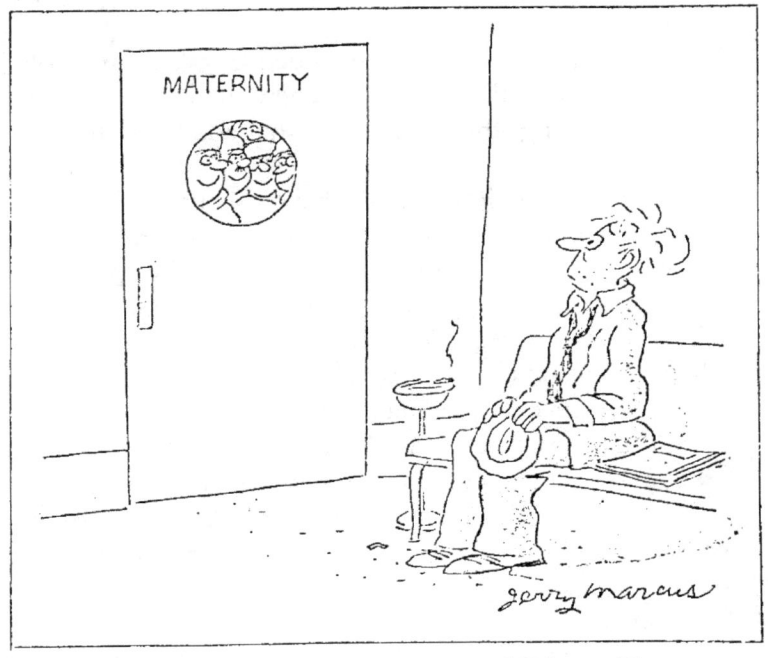

From Good Housekeeping, August 1976, p. 26
Used with permission.

Couvade (from the French word couver, meaning 'to hatch') is the custom which required the husband of the woman who is giving birth to lie in bed and fast from eating certain foods. In some cultures he would moan and groan as though he were experiencing the discomforts of giving birth and then he would receive the solicitous attention of his female relatives.

This custom, or a variation of it, has been found in all parts of the world. Anthropologists have discovered the practice of <u>couvade</u> in such diverse locations as China, India, Africa, the East Indies, in certain of the Baltic provinces, and the Americas.

Surprising as it may seem, our Space Age specialists are the neo-primitives when it comes to childbirth. They show no consideration for the father-to-be. The only role they assign to a new father is that of bringing flowers to his wife the day after she has delivered and paying the hospital bill upon her discharge.

In Russia the husband is accorded an even lesser role in his wife's childbirth experience. There, he cannot even visit his wife during the nine days she and her infant are hospitalized.

Though Americans may have slipped behind the Russians in the exploration of outer space, they have maintained a slim superiority over them in the appreciation of childbirth and its effect upon the inner space of the human mind. Nevertheless, there is no room for smugness. There is still much to be done yet in the United States in order to achieve fully-humanized childbirth.

If today's husbands' needs at the moment of childbirth are not effectively met, it is not that they have not made an effort to reveal their yearnings. Husbands have been communicating their needs regarding childbirth. However, their audiences have been inattentive and, accordingly, they have missed the message.

Take the matter of play, for example. Much is revealed by the way one behaves while playing.

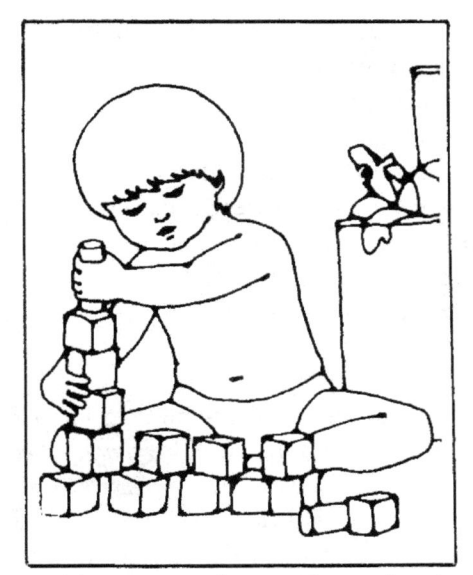

For a child, play is not just a way of killing idle hours. In play a child can rearrange things to better suit himself. He may not actually own a pony, but in play he can gallop to his heart's content.

In play a child can reinforce what he already knows. With blocks he can build a house, starting with the ground and working up to the roof, putting in the door just where it should be, and the chimney, too.

But most of all, play is a self-validating experience. As a child crawls over furniture, climbs up stairs, and struggles to maneuver with his father's shoes on, he is inwardly saying, "I can do it! I am able, and no one can say I'm not."

Probably the most characteristic form of play for a father to engage in with his toddler is throwing the youngster into the air and catching the laughing, squealing child as it drops into his arms. President John F. Kennedy was caught by the cameraman in many charming poses with his children; one of them was of him tossing Caroline into the air and catching her in the backyard of the home the Kennedys occupied while he was a Senator.[4]

The sorrow of a father no longer able to play in this manner with his child was poignantly expressed by George Lathrop, after the death of his only child:

The Child's Wish Granted

Do you remember, my sweet absent son,
How in the soft June days forever done

You loved the heavens so warm and clear and high:
And when I lifted you, soft came your cry -
"Put me way up – way up in the blue sky."

I laughed and said I could not - put you down
Your gray eyes filled with wonder beneath that crown
Of bright hair gladdening me as you raced by.
Another Father now, more strong than I,
Has borne you voiceless to your dear blue sky.[5]

Colman mentioned this unique father-child mode of interaction in *Pregnancy: The Psychological Experience*. He wrote, "Impending fatherhood uncovers all the memories and emotions of what it was like to be fathered as a child. Father-to-be may be flooded by forgotten images - playing ball, being tossed in the air, doing household repairs together..."[6]

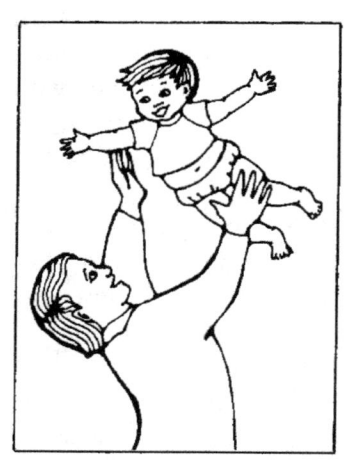

Playing ball and doing house-hold repairs together are not activities mothers generally engage in with their sons, and neither is tossing them into the air and catching them. On the contrary, mothers are usually fearful on seeing the ritual performed.

It is the typical, fatherly way of playing with his young child, however, and for a father to catch his child in mid-air is as self-validating for him as any play engaged in by a child. "I can do it!" is the silent cry of a father as he extends his hands to catch his child.

A father should not be restrained from catching his child until the youngster is a toddler, however. There is no better time for a father to catch his child than at the moment of that infant's birth.

Neil Collins recounted the change in his attitude toward homebirth which occurred during his wife's second pregnancy. He voiced satisfaction when he spoke of the many emotional changes which he went through until he began to think in terms of "wouldn't it be nice if we could have our baby in our own bedroom."[7]

"Over the past six months my thoughts had evolved from 'Of course not!' through 'I hope not' into 'Oh dear!' to 'Sure' and finally to 'I can.'"

Any father can personally receive his child at the moment of birth. Furthermore, it is good for him to do so.

Doctors are slowly becoming aware that a husband has something to gain by actively participating in his wife's childbirth experience. It is for this reason that Dr. Bradley encourages the new father to take pictures of his wife and baby immediately after the birth.[8] He says this gives the husband "a feeling of usefulness." Other activities conceded to a husband in the labor and delivery rooms (by those doctors who permit natural childbirth) are sponging the wife's face with a damp face cloth, rubbing her back and offering her a lollipop to suck.

The limitations of the above as satisfactory vehicles of interaction between man and wife were illustrated in a childbirth film that was popular a few years back, entitled "The Story of Eric." While his wife was on the delivery table, the young father did change the face cloth on her forehead, and did put his arm around her back to raise her up during a contraction. It was the doctor, however, to whom the young woman looked at the end of each contraction. It was the doctor with whom she exchanged smiles. It was the doctor who told her she was doing 'great.' He even rested his hand on her leg at one point. During all this, the young husband was reduced to the role of a minor functionary.

In a magazine article about a midwest doctor who does home deliveries, there was a picture of a mother in labor looking up at her doctor and the caption read, "Though it is mostly unspoken, there is definitely dialogue between doctor and mother."[9]

It is the husband who should have the principal role in the corporeal dialogue at this moment in the love life of the couple. No third party was needed nine months earlier when conception occurred. At the moment of childbirth, when a woman is making her response to the genital gesture her man had initiated, no one should come between them then, not even briefly.

The husband of the woman in the above article sensed the inadequacy of the role assigned to him when birth was imminent and the doctor handed him a face cloth, saying, "Mop her brow."

Rebelling inside himself, the father wrote, "But this is not YOUR role in this. It comes when she grasps your hand, tenderly this time, and you know she wants you to share in her ultimate triumph." But if the baby has been born, caught by someone else, it is too late to truly share in her moment of exaltation.

In an article entitled "Diary of an Expectant Father," the new father reports more than he realizes in describing the following delivery room scene:

> Then she [his wife, Susan] was bearing down again, the doctor's steady voice urging her on. I glanced down to the foot of the delivery table, where, beyond the sterile sheet that covered Susan's abdomen, the obstetrician and the resident were crouching. "Two more good ones, and we should have it," the doctor said. Susan clenched her teeth and pushed. There's the head!" the doctor exclaimed. "Now give me one more good one for the shoulders."
>
> Everyone in the room seemed to be pushing with her now, as Susan tensed her body for one last effort, and then a nurse called out, "It's a girl," and the doctor was holding up my daughter..."[10]

Notice the language - "Two more good ones, and we should have it." "Now give me one more good one."

[emphasis added]

With everyone pushing, including the father (no doubt with eyes closed and teeth clenched) it was the doctor who received this young woman's gift of love. He was the partner in this genital action of hers. In a hospital it can hardly be otherwise.

The same displacement can occur when a midwife assists at a homebirth. In *The Home Birth Book*, Lee Simon described her birth experience. Although her husband's arm was around her shoulders all the while it was the midwife who was the significant one in her life at that moment.

Lee said, in regard to the midwife, "We had a good working relationship. I felt we were integrated in our efforts. When I hesitated, Jan's voice came through clear and direct...It was a tremendous feeling to trust someone like that when I needed support and concentration."[11]

Later Lee did state she could not have given birth without the help of her husband, Phil. Nevertheless, by her own admission, it was the midwife on whom she primarily depended during the experience of birth.

When a doctor or midwife steps in between husband and wife at childbirth and receives the woman's love gift, the relationship between husband and wife suffers. Their focus of attention is on that third person. What he, or she, is doing becomes of primary concern, and man and wife, momentarily, forget each other.

They forget each other, too, in the hospital when a fetal monitor is being used. A *New York Times Magazine* article described this distraction as experienced by one couple. Mrs. Phillips was in the labor bed and was "hooked up to a machine." Her husband was sitting in a chair beside the bed. "Within seconds, Mr. and Mrs. Phillips were intently watching two moving lines on a television-like box beside the bed. Throughout the early hours of her labor...Mrs. Phillips watched the gray metal box with its dials and meters, oscilloscope and blinking lights."[12] Subtly, the psychic energy of man and wife was diverted from each other.

A similar distraction occurs when a woman bottle-feeds her infant instead of breastfeeding her. In breastfeeding, a mother just holds her infant close and puts her nipple into the child's mouth. She relaxes and enjoys the infant's presence while the baby discovers the rewards of her own efforts as she gets her belly filled. Neither knows nor cares about the temperature of the milk, the rate of milk flow, nor the length of time the interaction will require. United in a tender bond, time stops for the two of them and the relationship is all they know.

The following poem captures the nursing experience:

My Baby's Hand

Velvet soft, my baby's hand -
A feather floats across my chest
And lands upon my other breast
Exploring.
Restless yet, my baby's hand -
A spider leaves its silken bed
To dance in space upon a thread
Soaring.
Reaching now, my baby's hand -
A snowflake falls upon my lips
Shaped like tiny finger tips
Adoring.
Still at last, my baby's hand -
As dreams begin to be unfurled
The two of us, all the world
Ignoring.

Dorothy Roberts

When a mother uses a bottle, instead of breastfeeding her baby, their relationship is sacrificed for an object. The focus of attention of both mother and child is not on each other but on the intervening object, the bottle.

The mother is concerned that the milk is the right temperature. She must remember to hold the bottle at the correct angle so that the nipple is full of milk, and not air. She must be certain that the milk is flowing at the right speed. It should not flow too fast, yet must be fast enough so that the baby does not get tired from the struggle and go to sleep before she is through with her feeding.

The baby, too, concentrates on the bottle-object. Before long her little hands rest on it, instead of reaching up to touch mother's face, tug her hair, or playfully spear her nostrils.

Eventually, mother discovers that the baby is more comfortable lying down in her crib or playpen holding her own bottle. All mother is required to do is to fill it. Thus, a significant, tender, touch relationship eludes them.

A similar rift occurs when the birthing couple permits a third party with or without a monitor to come between them at the moment of childbirth. The attention of both is shifted from each other to the interloper. How many contractions will it take until it is all over? Will the doctor have to cut? Is it a boy or a girl? These become the principal concerns of husband and wife as their relationship is sacrificed on the altar of the delivery table.

Roy V. Boedeker, M.D., a St. Louis obstetrician, extolling the episiotomy, a small cut to facilitate the expulsion of the baby's head during birth, said, "We inject a little novocaine, make a little cut, lift the baby out gently with forceps, then repair and restore the pelvic floor even better than God made it."[13] That may be so, but it is a shame a love relationship would be destroyed just to preserve a pelvic floor.

The relationship remains intact when the couple gives birth in the dimly-lit seclusion of their bedroom, with each person yielding to the hidden forces of love. As one young father said, "You discover strengths you never knew you had."

Dorothy V. Whipple, M.D., made an interesting statement regarding the development of a woman.

Declaring that bottle feeding a baby is a little like getting pregnant by artificial insemination, she explained, "Both these modern techniques produce results, in the one case a well-nourished baby, in the other a pregnancy. But Nature has designed other ways of accomplishing these goals, the experiencing of which can contribute to personality development."[14]

Present hospital delivery practices could also be included in this analogy. Obstetric techniques are effective in getting a baby out of his mother's abdomen, but for personality development of husband and wife, Nature has designed a different way.

In giving birth a woman is making a corresponding gesture to the one her beloved had made nine months earlier. Just as it was appropriate and rewarding for her to be present and participating in his genital expression so in childbirth it is equally fitting for her man to be present and participating in hers. If approached in the same manner as coitus was, with kisses and caresses and the lights turned down, birth will be exquisitely rewarding for husband as well as wife, with no undue strain on mother's pelvic floor.

In the *Ascent of Man*, J. Bronowski wrote, "The march of man is the refinement of the hand in action...It is the hand that drives the subsequent evolution of the brain."[15]

The hand of a husband is primed for achieving the ultimate in creative expression as his wife's pregnancy progresses. Feeling the baby kicking inside his wife's body puts a man in touch with his child and is reassuring for him. When, at long last, in the seclusion of their bedroom he is permitted to give his wife perineal massage and support and to coax his child from her body with his own hands, he will discover and truly know that "she is indeed bone of my bone, and flesh of my flesh." And he will at last experience that peace for which he has yearned for so long.

Irrevocable damage is done to a man when he is prevented from personally receiving his wife's gift of love at the moment of childbirth. When birth is experienced as a genuine husband/wife love encounter, as it was intended to be, dignity and life are restored to a man and a new tomorrow made possible.

MARILYN A. MORAN

6. DOCTOR'S DILEMMA

At this point in the discussion obstetricians have probably broken out in a collective case of the hives from the thought of the dire consequences of women trying to give birth at home without their expert assistance. What these men have lost sight of is the fact that women have been faultlessly designed to give birth by an all-provident Creator. Down through the millennia they have been doing it, moreover, with obvious success.

"My ways are not your ways." The ways and means of couples giving birth at home are not the ways employed by doctors in delivering a baby, and they should not be. The techniques of doctors are too restrictive. Furthermore, in many instances, they are counter-productive to a safe and easy birth.

The tools used by today's couples in giving birth at home are the techniques of lovemaking, and they are highly effective in accomplishing the desired end, with minimum discomfort and maximum satisfaction for both husband and wife. The interconnection between the birth experience and the love relationship is charmingly revealed in many of the personal accounts in *Hey Beatnik!,* a book about the Stephen Gaskin Farm in Tennessee where the farm's own midwives have delivered over 1,000 babies at home.

In describing her birth experience, Pamela told of how her 'rushes' slowed down and the progress of labor just about halted. In talking with the midwives she confessed that when she and Wayne got married they left out of the service the part about "for better or worse, in sickness and in health, 'til death do us part" because Wayne objected to the phrase.

"So Stephen married us for real right there, made us repeat the vows, and I could feel a miracle happen. Five minutes later Christopher was born. He was all pink and hollering and looking around."[1]

Another episode, the story of Jean, contained a similar account of the connection between the birth and the love relation. This mother had been fully dilated for five hours, yet labor had made little progress. All of a sudden Jean's contractions became stronger. She had been thinking about how much she loved her husband, Leigh, and when she started to tell him so, the baby began to move down the birth canal. As Cara, one of the Farm midwives said, "Over and over again, I've seen that the best way to get a baby out is by cuddling and smooching with your husband. That loving, sexy vibe is what puts the baby in there, and it's what gets it out, too."[2]

All it takes is the stimulus of love for the laboring woman's cervix and perineum to yield. Failure to make use of the love-type aids for delivery can cause complications and distress. The intelligent thing to do is to utilize the natural faculties for birth. This is what the couples who give birth at home are doing with enviable success.

Massage of the perineum is one of the techniques which can be used by a husband as he assists his wife in giving birth. The perineum is the area between the vagina and anus. For centuries midwives have massaged this region with or without a lubricant such as olive oil, in order to keep the tissue soft and pliable during labor and birth.

In recent years the art of perineal massage and support has become popularized by Norman Casserley, a male midwife. He claims to have delivered 3,500 babies during the last twenty years without a single flesh tear by using this technique. According to him when the area is kept naturally flooded with blood by massage and the pelvic floor is relaxed, tearing will not occur and an episiotomy (a small incision) is not necessary. Casserley claims that manual manipulation of the vaginal area by experienced hands during passage of the head prevents tissue tears externally and internally.[3]

Others also are finding tactile stimulation effective for the woman in childbirth. *Newsweek* carried an article about an electrical vibrating device being used by a Swedish obstetrician, Dr. Sune Dahlgren. When the five-inch stainless steel rod is applied to the mother's cervix it causes such effective relaxation that the length of labor is usually cut in half. According to *Newsweek,* "The accounts of women on whom the vibrator has been tried have been so glowing that nearly every mother entering Eskilstuna Central Hospitals maternity unit is now demanding that it be used for her own deliveries...Mothers who have given birth before are thrilled with the difference."[4]

A husband need not hesitate to stimulate his wife's perineum during childbirth because he lacks Casserley's vast experience or Dahlgren's stainless steel vibrator. If he has been a tender, loving husband during the past nine months he has acquired all the experience necessary in the massage of his wife's perineum, and she has long since discovered how to yield to his touch.

Women find perineal massage and support by their husbands comforting and even pleasurable. Some also find delight in placing their own hand on the baby's advancing head, with their husband giving support from below. It is easy, especially with no nurse or doctor around to scold them about maintaining the 'sterile field.'

Another love-type aid in assisting a woman in childbirth which is available to a husband, but not to an obstetrician (unless he is her husband) is that maneuver called 'smooching.' It is quite effective in getting the mother's perineum to relax.

There is an intricate connection between the mouth and the birth canal. Margaret Camper, R.N., one of America's best-known childbirth educators, recommends yawning to encourage relaxation during labor as it helps one to let loose all over. She continues her instruction with the suggestion, "Part your lips in a faint Mona Lisa smile, just so the teeth and tongue are not touching. The tongue should rest loosely in your mouth, every muscle of your face should be relaxed."[5]

Sheila Kitzinger, the British childbirth educator, is equally explicit in her recommendations concerning the mouth at the moment of birth. She advises that as the baby approaches the perineum and slowly eases through the birth outlet, the mother should relax her lips, tongue and throat, and she should smile.[6]

When Frances Trute was giving birth in the hospital, her Lamaze 'monitrice' kept telling her, during contractions, to relax her face and mouth. However, because she was so overwhelmed with the strength of the contractions Frances said she had trouble remembering <u>where</u> her mouth was! Had she been 'necking' with her husband she would have experienced no such difficulty.

Besides contributing to the relaxation and gentle stretching of the perineum, smooching confers an additional benefit. It places man and wife in the <u>en face</u> position, which is just as essential in fostering interest and affection between man and wife as it is in fostering interest and affection between mother and child.

Many hospitals are now permitting husbands to be with their wives in the delivery room. However, the stipulation is generally made that the husband must remain seated on the anesthesiologist's stool, behind his wife's head or just slightly to the side. This positioning prevents an <u>en face</u> encounter between husband and wife. Therefore, it interferes with the bonding which is occurring between them.

Another little-known technique for a more gentle birth experience is breast and nipple stimulation. As many children have observed, dogs and cats lick their nipple area repeatedly while giving birth. It is generally assumed that this is done in the interest of cleanliness. However, the animal's self-licking of the nipple area serves a more important function than that. This tactile stimulation triggers the release of the hormone oxytocin, one of nature's provisions for a successful birth, as it causes the uterus to empty its contents.

And it is not only small mammals that use tactile stimulation of this part of the body during labor to effect the release of oxytocin. The practice has been found in certain human cultures as well. Margaret Mead and Niles Newton report that breast manipulation during labor is used by both the Lepcha people of Asia and the Siriono's of Bolivia.[7] Furthermore, breast manipulation during labor is frequently suggested by the midwives at the Stephen Gaskin Farm.

At the Midwives Conference in El Paso, Texas, in January 1977, Ina May Gaskin related a very interesting story about a unique adaptation of the customary use of breast stimulation. Labor, for a certain couple, had been quite prolonged. Ina May noticed there was very little touch used between husband and wife. Therefore, she suggested that the husband lie down in bed and the wife smooch with him and stimulate his nipples. The technique worked beautifully! According to the midwife, "...all at once the baby was just trying to get out. We barely got her back on the bed in time..."[8]

The midwives at the Stephen Gaskin Farm are not the only ones in this country to take note of the beneficial effects of breast stimulation during labor. In recent years many nursing mothers have discovered this provision of nature, without realizing it.

A few decades ago a nursing mother generally breastfed for three to six months, and then put her infant on a bottle. However, under the influence of the LaLeche League, a mother today frequently nurses until her youngster becomes disinterested in the breast. Many times this does not happen until the child is eighteen months of age, or even older. Sometimes it doesn't happen until the child is three years old.

As a result, many pregnant women have a toddler that still enjoys being nursed at naptime and again before going to bed at night. These mothers report that when they nurse their toddler during the early stage of labor, their contractions get much stronger.

One mother said that when she nursed her young son during labor she had to use her Lamaze breathing because the contractions became so strong. Adam thought it was fun having Mommy blowing in his face and on his hair. Needless to say, mother didn't share his glee!

It remains a mystery why more people are not aware of the effect of breast stimulation on the progress of labor. Granted, obstetricians cannot be expected to know of the latest craze among the commune crowd nor among those 'kookie' nursing women, let alone the habits of some tribe in a remote jungle of South America. Doctors should know what is being written in their own medical journals, however, and the subject of breast stimulation to induce labor has been discussed there.

Obstetrics & Gynecology carried an article by T. Vago, M.D. and A. Jhirad, M.D., in which they report on an experiment they conducted on 204 women. Labor was induced by the use of a breast pump which was operated by the mothers. The overall success rate was 69.6%.

The authors stated, "Breast stimulation activates endogenous oxytocin which results in physiologic uterine contraction...we strongly believe that in cases where [amniotomy or oxytocin] are contraindicated, breast stimulation should be used."[9]

Also, included in the proceedings of the Fourth World Conference of the International Federation of Gynecologists and Obstetricians, in 1964, was a report by R. E. Gadea, entitled, "New Methods for Induction of Labor: Breast Suction."[sic] So, the subject has been discussed in medical literature.

Furthermore, one obstetrician, the chief of the department of obstetrics and gynecology at a mid-western hospital, when questioned about the effect of breast stimulation on the progress of labor replied, "It is a well-known fact that nipple stimulation, whether by a baby or a breast pump, triggers some secretion of oxytocin and has been used to stimulate a lazy labor."

It may be a well-known fact among the medical profession, but it certainly has been a carefully guarded secret from the laity!

Marriage manuals all say, "Anything goes!" in the lovemaking between man and wife. The authors of those books did not have childbirth in mind. It is interesting to discover that those gestures which they did have in mind are fitting and effective in bringing the childbirth encounter to a rewarding climax, too.

In one study of home deliveries which were handled by midwives the consensus was reached that midwives should be permitted to administer pitocin (synthetic oxytocin) in the event of uterine inertia. With one's loving husband around "doing what comes naturally," however, uterine inertia should never develop.

H.O.M.E., in their instructions about controlling postpartum hemorrhaging state, "If it is possible to get the baby to nurse immediately, it will help in the release of oxytocin which helps the uterus to contract. If not, gentle massaging of the nipples of the breast may serve as a substitute."[10] It would seem, however, that if the couple had approached birth as an intimate encounter in marital love, the woman's circulatory system would already be awash with oxytocin, thus rendering concern about hemorrhaging unnecessary.

The above points are utterly extraneous to the experience of all but a few obstetricians. The majority of them have been so pre-occupied with the evacuation of the uterus that it has never occurred to them to take a good look beneath the drapery enshrouding the birthing woman. If they did look closely due north of that uterus in which they are so engrossed, they would discover a woman, a human being, making a human gesture and they would instinctively fade into the background, knowing they had intruded where they have no right to be.

One of the few men who have had the courage to look with both eye and mind at the laboring woman is William Hazlett, M.D., of Kingston, Pa. He has reflected upon birth and has adapted his method of assisting at birth to conform to what he has observed. Here is a sample of his insights in the matter:

> There are many gradients of husband participation at birth. The man can participate in fantasy at home or bar while immersing himself in alcohol. He can pace the waiting room. He can wait with his wife while continuous spinal anesthesia cloaks her labor and the obstetrician delivers the baby. He can work with her as she labors naturally and then on her removal to the delivery room, drop out. Or he can accompany her and work with her until the birth. The last seems infinitely better than the first. But must this be all?
>
> If he is so good at rubbing her back and directing the breathing and relaxation during the first stage of labor, then at the end why should he not also serve as midwife and deliver their child?
>
> Birth is qualitatively different when the husband participates in the natural birth, in contrast to the time before if he waited outside. Separately their bodies and minds unite, then unities strive to merge to create the larger unity. The husband as midwife simply goes one step farther to complete a unity which, sadly enough as one thinks about it, never can be so.
>
> To seek that impossible unity is still worth the struggle because to the wife or the husband who has succeeded in the accomplishment of their instinctive purpose comes self-esteem, a consolation prize of no small value; not only to each and to the unity-seeking couple, but also to others. For self-esteem is a catalyst to love and a feeling for justice toward

others, it serves to redirect human energies (human aggression, as the anthropologists would say) into creative and humanely constructive channels, and it counteracts our pernicious tendency to hate.[11]

Because of his insights regarding the beneficial effects of childbirth as a shared experience between husband and wife, if labor is proceeding normally and if the couple wishes, Dr. Hazlett actually permits the father to catch the baby. He stands by and acts as supervisor, while the parents do all the work themselves. He doesn't interfere unless needed.

The father's task is to support the baby's head in the palm of his hand as the mother eases it out. "Don't try to take the baby. Let her give it to you. Let her put it in your hands, "Hazlett wisely coaches."[12]

Dr. Hazlett has had about 400 couples give birth in this novel arrangement. One couple drove eighty miles from Chenango Bridge, N.Y. to have their baby the Hazlett way. Not only does he permit the father to catch the baby, but he also permits the mother to give birth in the labor room bed instead of being transferred to the delivery room. In the labor bed the mother can assume a more comfortable position for giving birth, as her legs are not elevated and in stirrups. In addition, the father is not required to don the traditional surgical dress, mask, and gloves.

Carolyn Butwin, one of Hazlett's patients, voiced the essence of the fully humanized childbirth experience when she spoke of "the symbolism of pushing out the baby to his father."[13]

Other couples who have given birth in the hospital with an obstetrician doing the actual catching of the baby claim to have fully shared the birth experience. They have been deluded. If all a husband is permitted to do is put a face cloth on his wife's forehead, or hand her a lollipop (the ultimate symbol of immaturity and incompetence), the best part has escaped him. To fully share the birth experience requires more husband-wife contact than that.

The language of love is touch. In the conjugal union it is touch of an intimate nature.

William Hazlett is the pioneer obstetrician in the humanization of childbirth as well as the hominization of man, to use a term which Hazlett has borrowed from Teilhard. Despite his intuitions about the importance of the childbirth experience in the growth and development of man and wife and despite the giant step he has taken in making it a more satisfying experience for them, the Hazlett way is still not the same as giving birth at home in a real love encounter manner. To begin with, he routinely gives the mother a mild sedative. If birth is experienced as a sexual encounter, that should hardly be required. The husband needed no mild sedative nine months earlier when impregnation occurred. His wife does not need one now, either, if the art of lovemaking is put to use completely.

But more important is the level of consciousness on which the husband experiences the birth of his child. With a third party standing by giving instructions it is too cerebral an event. A husband is not a pseudo-obstetrician. He is first and foremost a lover. He should be able to participate in the birth of his child on a level of deep and tender feelings, the same level on which he had participated when conception of the child occurred. Indeed he not only should, he <u>must</u> in order to receive the full benefit of the experience.

Because the sense of touch is heightened in the absence of vision, the dimly-lit seclusion of their own bedroom is the ideal environment for the birthing couple to interact most fully.

A young Kansas City couple gave birth at home with a doctor there to help. It was a long labor, so finally the doctor went ahead and did an episiotomy and delivered the baby, instead of letting the father receive his child. Although the young father never left his wife's side during the birth, and knew, intellectually, that his daughter had been born, afterwards he sensed that his wife was still having contractions. So he rushed into the room where she had labored as if to help her.[14] Intellectual knowledge is not enough. One must physically experience the act of love for the message to reach the core of one's being.

This is where obstetricians, even those who favor natural childbirth, make their mistake. They consider childbirth as something happening to a woman but have not realized that something is simultaneously happening to her man. He is as ready as she is for the experience and he yearns to participate in it fully.

In many childbirth manuals the husband is spoken of as a coach, a trainer who carefully watches, exhorts, and criticizes, while his wife conditions and learns to control her body during labor and delivery. Using this comparison Dr. Bradley states, "your duties as a husband and coach [are] to prepare your obstetrical athlete properly for the great event - labor and the birth of your child."[15] He even entitled his book *Husband-Coached Childbirth*.

The woman in childbirth is not swimming the English Channel! Rather, she is performing a cosmic dance, and it is not a solo performance. She is engaged in a pas de deux and her husband is her partner in the event. What he does, and does not do, affects her conduct, rendering it either spectacular or mediocre. By being lovingly sensitive to each others needs a husband can bring out the best in his wife, as she brings out the best in him. The moment of childbirth is their command performance, for which the two have long been waiting and preparing.

Although some obstetricians may concede that a homebirth is emotionally more rewarding than a hospital 'delivery,' the issue of safety invariably causes them to resist changing their minds on the subject. Years ago many women did die while giving birth from one of two causes, childbed fever or hemorrhage.

Childbed fever is due to lack of cleanliness during the birth or shortly thereafter. Those same precautions taken in the hospital today to avoid infection can be taken by the birthing couple at home.

Hemorrhage, as already noted, is avoided by putting the

baby to the breast immediately after birth. This stimulates the release of oxytocin which contracts the uterus, shutting off the open blood vessels. It is also avoided by not pulling on the cord to hurry the expulsion of the placenta. Obstetricians know of these safety precautions. Therefore, they are inclined to stress the danger to the child if birth takes place at home.

It is possible that a few babies with some genetic defect will die because their mothers gave birth at home where life-saving equipment was not readily available. Obstetricians tend to stress this point. But consider the fact that many of these same doctors have themselves ended the lives of millions of healthy babies through the practice of abortion. "Freedom of choice," the rallying cry of obstetricians in the last few years, is a two-edged sword and homebirth couples have now grabbed the handle.

Actually, birth at home is not as dangerous as couples have been led to believe. They have been misled into thinking that only professionals in a hospital are capable of assisting the woman in childbirth. The belief has been accepted without criticism throughout most of the technically advanced countries. It is time for couples, themselves, to examine the facts concerning the humanly art of childbirth, for it is they who have the most to gain, and the most to lose, by the manner in which it is experienced.

The Bible says, "A man shall leave his father and mother, and shall cleave to his wife: and they shall be two in one flesh." (Genesis 2:24) The moment of childbirth is an experience of this oneness, and is as much a time for closeness and intimacy as is the wedding night. In either event in-laws and doctors are only in the way.

This may seem difficult for obstetricians to accept at first, as it goes counter to what they have been taught. However, they have set a precedent for themselves when they shifted their attitude about abortion from one of opposition to one of acceptance and accommodation.

In April 1972 (nine months before the Supreme Court

decision liberalizing abortion laws) there appeared an article in the *American Journal of Obstetrics and Gynecology*. In it the authors, all professors of obstetrics at the leading medical schools across the country, discussed ways and means of providing for the one million abortions per year which they anticipated that would be requested of the medical profession. They admitted that to do abortions would be a change In the doctors traditional role of healer "but it will be necessary to make this change if we are to serve the new society in which we live" they stated.[16]

Well, the <u>new</u> "new society" has requests to make of obstetricians, also. These young women want prenatal care and back-up services from their doctors if they should decide to go to the hospital for assistance during or following a homebirth. If obstetricians will meet the requests of women seeking to destroy the innocent life within them, certainly they will be just as understanding toward those who seek to give their babies the very best.

But it is not just because they have been asked for certain services that the doctors will comply with the requests. Rather, obstetricians will provide prenatal care and back-up services to homebirth couples because it is right and just that they do so.

Women are human beings and deserve to be treated as such. They are not treated as persons in the standard hospital delivery situation. Women with a strong sense of personhood are crying out to have this fact recognized. They cannot go back to the old-fashioned way of giving birth again.

PART TWO

The Eyes Have Not Seen, Nor the Ears Heard…

7. THE ENERGY OF LOVE

> Love is the most universal, formidable, and mysterious of cosmic energies.
> Teilhard de Chardin

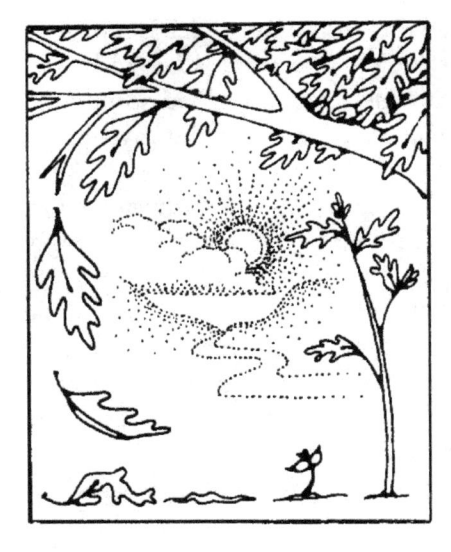

Man, despite his powers to perceive, his great curiosity, and his inventiveness, is still very much a child of creation. With his roots in biological life he is bound by the universal laws of life, one of which is that nature works inexorably in cycles. Man must not interfere with <u>any</u> of nature's cyclic patterns. Ecological collapse results when he does so.

Natural cyclic patterns are an integral aspect of every form of life, including the love-life of husband and wife. Married couples have been mindless of this fact. In order for the natural cycle of marital gift-giving to remain unbroken, childbirth must be fully experienced and fully shared by both members of the love dyad. When an obstetrician steps in between the lovers at the moment of birth to catch the baby, the cyclic giving and receiving of significant genital gifts is shattered.

There is nothing in the intellect which is not first learned through the senses. It is not enough that an obstetrician tell a man he has a fine, new son. It is not enough that a man see his child emerge from his wife's body. For a man to really be open to the action of love he must personally participate, with his own hands.

Human sex is an act of gift-giving. This is what distinguishes human sex from animal copulation. And it is also what distinguishes human birth from that experienced by animals. In coitus a man volitionally bestows upon his beloved his most precious gift, from which he relinquishes all possession. The cycle of gift-giving becomes complete at the moment of birth if the woman is able to personally give back to her beloved that which had originated with him nine months earlier, and to which she has added something of her own. This simple fact is the core of the mystery of marital love.

In coitus a man's action is centrifugal and the woman's action is centripetal. In childbirth the roles are simply reversed.

Helene Deutsch noted that a nursing mother's psychic energy flows outward toward her child with her stream of milk. In childbirth a woman's psychic energy is also flowing outward, this time with her child toward her husband, if he is the one sharing her personal space. As in breastfeeding, her action is centrifugal. But because childbirth has been misunderstood, the husband of the birthing woman has been unable to act centripetally and to become the receiver of her gift.

To interfere with the dynamics of marital love is as dangerous as tampering with any of nature's other cyclic systems. To impede a natural flow or to upset a natural balance is to invite ecological collapse. The eco-system of marriage is as susceptible to disruption as any other natural system.

Alienation, bickering, adultery, and battered children are but a few of the consequences of man's failure to realize that childbirth is a communication of love and a unifying force. The effects of disrupting this psychobioecosystem are impossible to avoid. It can be summed up in the Latin phrase <u>naturam expellas furca tarn en recurret.</u> You can drive nature out with a pitchfork; yet somehow she returns with a vengeance. Nature has been taking out her vengeance upon married couples and she will continue to do so, relentlessly, as long as they break her laws.

A husband needs to make contact with his beloved at the moment of childbirth. Love's great cycle must be allowed to reach completion if they are to achieve their destiny, and harness the energy of love.

> "It is possible for one person to love another and not have that love reciprocated; but complete love is a mutual exchange, a mutual sharing, accepting, union."
>
> Louis J. Lambert, S.J.

MARILYN A. MORAN

8. 21ST CENTURY GOTHIC

"Miracles spring from grace incarnate as normally as sparks from a fire."
Edward Schillebeeckx, O.P.

When the early Colonists arrived in this land 350 years ago, they found timbered forests, rolling grasslands, and clear-flowing streams and rivers. Being primarily farmers, these early settlers had only a minimal effect upon the countryside. They did clear some of the land for planting crops, and in time a scattering of villages and towns appeared throughout the wilderness.

It was not until this country changed from an agrarian nation to an industrial one, however, that the landscape became greatly altered. Rivers were dammed and reservoirs were created where once there had been green valleys. Pastures yielded to concrete jungles, and ribbons of asphalt eventually appeared lacing the countryside like streamers in a ticker-tape parade.

This new approach toward the land and its usefulness brought about the physical alterations. These changes were inevitable. It is part of the law of growth and development that when a change occurs in attitude and approach, a physical alteration takes place, too. When a man and woman in love change their attitude and behavior at the moment of childbirth, a change will be brought about in them, also.

Most women in the world give birth isolated from their husbands. During those rare instances when a husband is present he is treated as a minor functionary. This is the wrong approach entirely.

Today's society is characterized by alienation, marital discord, corruption and war. Childbirth as a love encounter, however, can do much to change all that. When a man personally receives his wife's gift of love, reconciliation is achieved and harmony established between them. As the fundamental discontent of marriage is eliminated, the prevalent social illnesses will gradually disappear like the morning fog before the advancing sun.

But when the bond between husband and wife is cemented, an even more concrete sign of their reconciliation will manifest itself. It is here proposed that when a man and woman communicate love to the complete satisfaction of the other, using childbirth as a genuine love encounter, run-away fertility will come to a halt.

This will occur because once the final goal of experiencing a fully-ratified love relationship is attained, any further need for fulfillment will subside. When this need subsides, so shall fertility.

These are strong statements to make. It would be nice if one could point to an obscure race or culture in which this phenomena occurred. This writer cannot. But it does stand to reason that once nature has reached an intended goal, further strivings would be unnecessary.

This could very well be due to the principle of opposing forces. Childbirth allows a perfect balancing between the forces of marital genital giving and receiving. When a man is permitted to receive with his own hands his wife's gift of love at the moment of birth, his ability to donate love's gift becomes balanced by his ability to receive love's gift. The same becomes true for his wife; her ability to receive, in coitus, becomes balanced by her ability to give, at the moment of childbirth.

In nature there are many instances of opposing forces being balanced with the same result occurring in each case -

a cancellation effect. For example, when the crest of a water wave meets the trough of another, the result is calm water. The same is true for sound waves, with the result being silence. For light waves the result is darkness.

Even a 'back yard' demonstration of this principle can be found. When two children on a swing-set swing in unison, the front legs of the swing-set tend to rise up as the children swing backward. And the back legs lift when the children swing forward. However, if one child starts to lag behind and is swinging forward as the other is swinging back, the opposing swings balance each other, and the lifting of the legs is eliminated, much to the relief of a mother who may be watching from afar.

Balancing the opposing love forces of donation and reception by placing them in juxtaposition will yield the same result for the energy of love as has been recorded for any other form of energy, i.e., a cancellation effect.

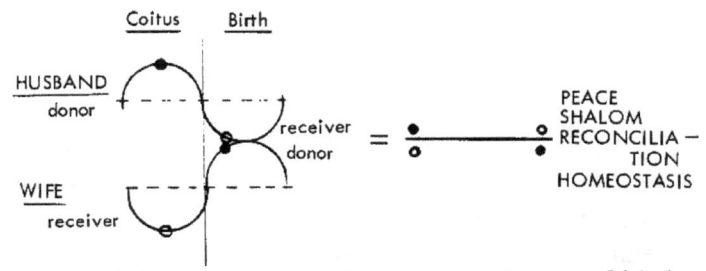

So, a "sufficiently secure basis for a regulation of birth, founded on the observance of natural rhythms" (*Humanae Vitae*, #24) may in fact exist.

Just as the butterfly sheds the cocoon from which it had emerged and no longer needs, and the baby gets rid of his umbilical cord and placenta when such organs are no longer useful, so too, when a husband receives back his gift of love in an experiential manner, conception will not occur again soon because the need to achieve receivership will no longer exist. Organic activity is goal-directed. When the goal has been achieved the activity wanes.

When it comes to childbirth, man has been guided more by culturally-induced fears than by his own instincts and needs. In his ignorance, he has disrupted the exquisite mechanisms of nature, much to his detriment. When couples do learn to approach childbirth as a genuine love encounter, and thereby cement their marital union, the effects of their goal-attainment will become evident.

Union is the critical word here. Embryologist Robert Francoeur defines union as "the arrangements of elements or monads in a synthesis which gives the participants a higher and new level of consciousness as well as a higher degree of complexity."

For too long the elements in the conjugal love dialogue (husband and wife) have been culturally deprived of the synthesis experience. Instead of being fused into a new, higher, and more complex level of consciousness (hormonal as well as psychic) man and wife have been permitted only to brush against each other fleetingly in coitus and then to drift apart as lonely and as empty as before. As a consequence man has found himself at an evolutionary dead end, arrested at an immature level of development and cut off from that higher degree of consciousness which is his due.

A new existence is possible, however. All a couple has to do is to change its attitude toward the birth experience.

Exactly what the mechanisms are which will be operating for those couples who do attain reconciliation, with its bonus of homeostasis, this writer cannot say with much certainty. What we are going to see is a situation similar to the appearance of the Gothic cathedrals in the twelfth and thirteenth centuries.

Prompted by their love of God and the Blessed Mother, saints and sinners, princes and peasants all combined their energies to fashion spectacular monuments of stone and glass unlike anything seen before or since. Bronowski spoke of the "audacity" of those builders for constructing such magnificent works, without even having the means for calculating the stresses involved. The people would just decide to build a beautiful church, and then they would do it. Each edifice became more spectacular than the one before.

The early Roman architects had no idea what jewels of construction the Gothic builders would eventually produce by abandoning the older form of architecture. Neither do today's obstetricians suspect what tomorrow's lovers will accomplish with the birth experience. But it is imperative that couples abandon the doctors' quasi-pathological approach to birth.

Incidentally, it was the careful balancing of opposing forces which permitted the construction of the Gothic cathedrals. By meeting thrust with counter-thrust, the builders overcame the limitations of Roman construction and higher vaults, lighter walls, and magnificent glass windows were free to emerge.

Man can build with stone and steel, but it remains for woman to construct the human dimension.

The freedom to produce new and remarkable achievements will be granted to those couples courageous enough to use their bodies to the fullest in the communication of love. All it will take is action at the moment of childbirth, triggered by mutual concern, empathy, respect and faith. Then the opposing forces of maleness and femaleness will be brought into harmony, and the new and balanced state of sexual integration (intra-personal as well as inter-personal) will be achieved. An added dividend can be foreseen when couples change in this way their approach to the childbirth experience. That extra something is nature's built-in control of the human population.

MARILYN A. MORAN

9. MUSINGS OF A NON-SCIENTIST

Nature has provided all species of life with built-in population controls. It seems, therefore, that man too should be so provided, without having to rely on chemical or mechanical contrivances, abortion, sterilization or homosexuality.

There is evidence that nature did not intend men and women to reproduce excessively. To begin with, there are relatively few days during the whole year that an individual woman is biologically fertile.

A girl does not start ovulating until her teen years and her ability to conceive a child ceases about thirty years later when her estrogen level drops. All told, her reproductive years are less than one-half her total life span.

There are also many factors which can affect a woman's ability to conceive. Thoughts and emotions have a great effect upon the workings of the human body, and this is especially true in regard to reproduction. Some women, wanting very much to become pregnant and yet unable to conceive, have developed a condition known as pseudocyesis. The symptoms are a cessation of both ovulation and menstruation plus a bloating of the abdomen similar to that which occurs during pregnancy.

Other women, unable to conceive a child, have adopted one only to discover a few months later that they are pregnant. Apparently, once they become confident regarding the task of mothering they are able to relax enough for conception to occur.

Anthropologists have reported some cultures in which there are no restrictions concerning premarital sex. Curiously enough, there are very few instances of conception occurring before marriage, although no preventative measures are taken. It seems the young people of those cultures engage in sexual relations just for a good time. And that is all they get out of it.

Conversely, studies reveal that in Western cultures many young unwed mothers actually wanted to get pregnant. Furthermore, the young men in question wanted to get them pregnant. They, too, got their hearts' desire.

Agnes deMille, the noted choreographer, made an interesting disclosure concerning dancers and their sexual development. Ballerinas are considered the epitome of femininity. However, they usually are flat-breasted and have small, boyish-looking hips. According to deMille, "Certain great soloists have been lacking in even primary sexual functions and are known to have menstruated rarely."

Apparently, as these women strive for perfection in their art in the process they unconsciously repress normal physiological development. The sequence of events permitting them to grow into women is disrupted, thereby curtailing their reproductive capacity and their real femininity.

Another instance of the relationship between the mind of a woman and her ability to conceive concerns what happens when she is raped. If the woman is genuinely violated she will spontaneously menstruate, regardless of which day of her menstrual cycle it is.

If a negative experience can alter the usual monthly cycle of a woman, a positive one can alter her reproductive cycle as well. There is no more positively satisfying experience than childbirth as a husband/wife love encounter.

Despite the many examples of the influence of the mind and heart in the matter of ovulation and reproduction, it will be found that nature's built-in control of the human population (via childbirth as a love encounter) actually has a biological basis. A few possibilities for this basis will be suggested.

Light affects the reproduction of many species of life, both plant and animal. Not only is light itself necessary, but the spectral range and the time at which exposure takes place also affect the reproductive outcome.

The composition of the light from incandescent bulbs differs greatly from the spectral range of sunlight. Because man has not evolved physiologically beyond the point he reached 10,000 years ago, when he had no supplementary light, he may be subjecting himself to unknown effects with his use of artificial light.

To use light which differs in spectral composition from daylight to the extent that Western man does is to repeatedly subject the human body to phototherapy. According to Richard J. Wurtman, who is an authority on the biological effects of light, "The findings already in hand suggest that light has an important influence on human health, and that our exposure to artificial light may have harmful effects of which we are not aware." During childbirth, that critical period of physiological reorganization, the judicious use of artificial light might be highly advisable.

Light plays a role in the human reproductive cycle, through its effects upon the pineal gland. Airline stewardesses on transoceanic flights (which shorten or lengthen their daylight hours) are notorious for menstrual irregularities. Other women with consistently irregular menstrual cycles have had them regularized by introducing additional illumination during the fourteenth through sixteenth nights of their cycle. Also, blind girls reach their menarche earlier than those with normal vision. So, there is indeed a connection between light and human reproduction.

Most non-induced births take place at night. It is possible that nature intended that little or no light reach the eyes of the human birthing couple at this critical period in their life. To give birth in the dark, or possibly by the light of one candle, may be very important in capitalizing upon nature's mechanism for control of the human population.

Smell is another factor to consider in studying reproduction. Pheromones are airborne chemical messengers from one organism to another which have a specific effect upon a target organ.

Insects use pheromones in trail-marking, alarm sounding, and in mating. So instrumental are these substances in mating behavior that synthetic pheromones are now being manufactured for use in the control of insect pests by luring the males to a trap.

Olfaction plays a role in the reproductive behavior of mammals, too. Female mice housed together away from any male will cease to ovulate. When they are exposed to the smell of even a few drops of male urine, however, their cycles resume.

A similar situation occurs with the rhesus monkey. If the male has its nostrils plugged with gauze he will show no interest in the presence of a sexually receptive female. When the plugs are removed, however, he quickly reveals acute awareness of the female's sexual state.

Humans also respond, unconsciously, to scents. Research reveals that a woman is highly sensitive to odor at the time of ovulation and progressively less so as the time of menstruation approaches. One researcher found that college girls housed together had their menstrual cycles synchronized, presumably through the mechanism of olfaction.

Apparently buried deep within humans is a communication system based upon smell. There may be extraordinary uses for this system that are as yet undiscovered. When a couple gives birth as a love encounter in the seclusion of their bedroom, and the husband finds it completely satisfying, it is not too farfetched to suggest that henceforth he might give off a new smell-print, one gonadally non-stimulating to his wife. This could very well be nature's biological pathway for bringing to a halt automatic, periodic ovulations.

Another factor relevant to this discussion is touch. There are some messages in this life that can be adequately transmitted either verbally or visually. But as for love and caring, they are best communicated through the sense of touch.

The father of the Prodigal Son could have just called out a greeting to the young man as he returned home. But by "throwing himself upon the neck" of the boy, he conveyed far more effectively his intense joy upon their reunion.

The need of a baby for human touch is well-documented. Despite adequate nourishment infants have been known to fail to thrive and eventually to die, in the absence of human touch. Youngsters deprived of affection and stunted in their growth have been placed in a loving environment and have started a growth spurt only to have it halt when they were returned to their former, loveless home.

Who can say adults are any less starved for touch? Who can say the touch of one's beloved at the moment of birth will have no biological effect? The importance of touch continues throughout life.

Another variable, and the last one to be suggested here, is lactation, which has a well-documented effect in producing a halt in periodic ovulations. Less well-known is its role in marital intimacy. Volumes have been written about the importance of breastmilk for a new baby, but scarcely a word has been written about its importance for a new father.

The *LaLeche League News* did print an article entitled "Sex and Breastfeeding" which dealt with this subject. Speaking of the confusion which some women have regarding the oftentimes pleasurable sensations accompanying lactation and the marital difficulty this can cause, the author wrote "some feelings of jealousy might be justified for men with wives who feel that pregnancy makes their bodies untouchable, or that lactation makes their breasts properly relegated to their babies alone. It doesn't."

Lactation can be an occasion of increased intimacy between husband and wife, enriching their relationship. This theme was illustrated in a beautiful painting by Veronese, one of the great masters of the 16th century. In his "Mars and Venus United by Love" Veronese shows a somewhat modestly draped Venus standing as Mars kneels on one knee before her. His left calf and hers are being tied with a pink ribbon by a diminutive cupid. Handsome Mars has his head turned away from Venus and is gazing out toward the viewer with a very thoughtful expression on his face. As he does so Venus is daintily expressing a few drops of milk from her right breast.

In the background another cupid, holding a golden sword, is restraining a magnificent, powerful horse. A guidebook of the Metropolitan Museum of Art (in which museum this painting now hangs) in its description of this painting states that the horse is a symbol of 'base passion,' which is here being restrained. It is via the lactating breast that it happens, if used as an instrument of marital love.

So, the role of lactation as a unitive force between man and wife may not be talked about very much, but it has been thought about, and for hundreds of years.

Generally, when a nursing mother arrives home from the hospital she has an uneasy suspicion that she is waist up for her baby, and waist down for her man. However, scripture states, "What God has joined together let no man tear asunder." By and large the lactating mother is a woman torn in two directions, unnecessarily.

If birth can be a bonding event, lactation can be too. Further-more, the discovery about oneself which occurred during the love encounter of birth could be reinforced through lactation, with the woman again being the donor of love's gift and her man once more experiencing that receivership which is so important to him.

Buckminster Fuller has stated that the flow of energy through a system tends to organize the system. When the energy of love is permitted to run its course unrestrained, it too will display highly-refined organization, to everyone's amazement.

It is very possible that part of this organization will be the halt of runaway fertility. Women who have learned to respond joyfully to their men not only on their wedding night but nine months later as well just might discover that they have no need of pills, nor coils, nor calendars.

Robert Ardrey has shown that when an animal has defended its territory successfully, it emerges a biologically superior specimen. The territory of the human pair-bond is their bedroom. When husband and wife have defended this territory successfully from disturbing cultural intrusions, they will emerge as superior specimens of the human race.

These superior specimens, united in a fully-consummated marriage, will be gifted with the supremely potent energy of love and will have the power to shape a new destiny for themselves and society. Nothing happens by chance in nature. Law governs all.

10. COVENANT OF LOVE

When couples ask counselors for help in achieving happiness in marriage they are invariably told to keep the channels of communication open. "Keep talking" is the advice they receive.

Talking is the tool for individuals interacting on a verbal level, but the fundamental discontent in marriage is not due to a breakdown in verbal communication. Discontent in marriage is caused by a failure to achieve communion on a much deeper level. Marriage concerns bodies, not tongues. The breakdown in verbal communication which occurs is only a symptom of a problem; it is not the problem itself. Unless couples can reach the core of the trouble, a truly harmonious marriage is impossible to achieve.

In marriage a man and woman enter a corporeal covenant - a covenant of flesh. An examination of what a covenant actually is will disclose an important mistake that most couples make. It is interference with the ritual enactment of the marriage covenant that makes the promised life of love and harmony impossible to achieve.

A covenant is a solemn agreement between two people, or two groups of people. It creates a relationship of mutual trust and fidelity which is unbreakable. In establishing a covenant both parties pledge certain actions, and both must participate in the ritual enactment which seals the agreement. Unlike a mere contract, a covenant establishes an artificial blood kinship between the parties.

The historical example is Sinai, where Yahweh promised the Israelites that He would be their God, and assist them and to deliver them to the Promised Land. The duties and obligations of the Israelites were to worship no other God but Yahweh, in the manner he prescribed, and to accept certain standards of conduct and morality as set forth in the Ten Commandments.

For the covenant ritual an altar was built and animals were sacrificed. One half of the blood of the animals was splashed on the altar, which represented Yahweh. After the terms of the covenant were read to the people and they accepted them the remaining blood was splashed on them.

Had the Israelites neglected to splash their bodies with the blood of the sacrificial animals, the covenant would be lacking their full participation in the ritual enactment. Without the necessary sign of ratification on their part, the covenant with Yahweh would have been devoid of power. For a covenant to have force, it is of the essence that both parties be present and both parties actively participate in the ritual enactment. Mere vocal consent is not enough.

In the covenant of marriage a woman is invited to participate intimately in the life of her husband. Her chance to truly take part in the ritual enactment of the love pledge is in the uniquely human experience of childbirth as a love encounter.

Like Israel, each bride is called to make the acceptable gift to her bridegroom. The action of a woman is no less important than that of a man in sealing their covenant relationship. A marriage is not valid unless both parties give consent. Similarly, a marriage is not a graced covenant unless both parties participate actively in its enactment. Partial participation is not enough.

The modern idea of sex for recreation but not procreation, mixed as it is with a lingering Victorianism regarding bodily functions, especially feminine ones, has obscured the sexual nature of pregnancy and birth. Yet, by all logic, the act of conception should proceed to a moment of great triumph and intense romance. And it is at this moment that the covenant of marriage is fully sealed.

As a husband coaxes his baby from his wife's body with his own hands, he will personally discover, "This one, at last, is bone of my bone and flesh of my flesh." With kinship established between them, understanding and harmony will be theirs, for it is Yahweh Himself, the God of love, who guarantees the covenant of marriage.

11. TO FEMINISTS AND FRIENDS

The story is told of Thomas Edison that once when he was busily engaged in one of his many experiments he tested 5000 possible combinations without accomplishing what he was trying to do. Someone commented, "What a shame. All that work, and no progress."

Undismayed, Edison replied, "Not at all. I now know 5000 things not to do."

From the presentation so far it should be evident that there are many things that couples, too, should not do if they are to achieve their goal of peace and harmony. The first thing to be avoided, if at all possible, is giving birth in the hospital with a doctor delivering the baby. (Of course, if the couple went to a hospital and the doctor and nurses stood outside the labor room door and let mother and dad have an intimate experience by themselves, that would be different. And there have been some cases in recent months of exactly that happening.)

The second act to be avoided is abortion. It is absurd for a woman to be on the verge of becoming reconciled with her man only to squander the opportunity by destroying her developing gift of love.

According to the law of social exchange, a stable peer relationship is maintained if one gives a gift to another and the receiver repays the debt with a gift of equal value. However, if the receiver fails to reciprocate, a shift occurs in the peer relationship. Then the gift-giver assumes a subtly superior or dominant position and the recipient is assigned an inferior or subordinate one. Furthermore, they both know it.

The only way to prevent this power shift from developing is for the receiver to make an adequate return of gifts or services to the original donor. When this happens trust is maintained. Generally, the intensity of the relationship then diminishes leaving good feelings in its wake.

In the conjugal social exchange coitus must be followed by childbirth as a love encounter in order to maintain the peer relationship. For a woman to have an abortion is to render herself unable to reciprocate with her genital gift of love. Choosing an abortion is choosing to remain in a relationship thrown far off-balance. The woman who makes such a choice locks herself into a position of inferiority in the eyes of her man, the very state which the women of today so violently abhor.

In his inimitable way Art Buchwald mentioned the importance of reciprocity in the law of social exchange. He had been thanking a Canadian friend for the brave deed the Canadians performed in smuggling some American diplomats out of Iran during the hostage crisis. In declaring there was no need for the Americans to thank the Canadians, his friend George explained, "You Americans don't really understand what makes another nation feel good. For years you people have been going around the world aiding other countries…No self-respecting country enjoys being on the receiving end of someone else's largesse. By doing something for you we have restored our national pride…For years Canadians have been in America's debt and frankly it's been a pain in the [neck.] For the first time we don't feel inferior to you."

That which is true regarding international relations is just as true regarding interpersonal relations. If women are tired of being made to feel inferior to men, then they too must take the initiative when the opportunity presents itself. It is the only way they will ever get to enjoy the satisfaction of being free of indebtedness to their men.

So, clearly, abortion does not serve the best interests of feminists. On the contrary, abortion and sexual equality are utterly incongruent. The act of abortion destroys a woman's chance for growth, reconciliation, and equality with her man and indirectly with all men. For if sexual equality is not established in the bedroom, it is not going to be realized anywhere.

Now the question might be asked, "What of the pregnant woman who is not married and not even certain which man is responsible for her pregnancy? In her case there is no relationship in need of reconciliation. Indeed, there is no relationship at all."

If a man and woman are not ready to engage in the reciprocal exchange of meaningful gifts, if they are not ready to engage in the ultimate bonding activity, they should not be sleeping together.

A thinking person will modify his behavior according to the appropriateness of the time. When a boy sees a girl with whom he would like to enter into an affectional bond he does not run up and immediately start hugging her. Rather he bides his time until it is appropriate, going through the preparatory smiling, speaking and hand-holding sequence of behavior first.

If the time does not seem right to advance to the next stage in bonding, then prudence is exercised. That is, if it seems that the young lady may not be ready to reciprocate with a smile, a conversation, or hand-holding, fear of disappointment causes the young man to refrain from initiating the action at that moment.

The same reasoning is valid as a guide to interpersonal behavior on a more intimate level. A woman's reciprocal response to a man in the love act is for her to come forth with her gift nine months later. It is what a man desires and is searching for. But if the couple is not ready for the act in its <u>entirety</u>, for the woman's gift as well as the man's, then they should postpone that activity until a more propitious moment. Love is a dialogue, not a monologue.

When young men and women understand what constitutes a woman's response to coitus, and the importance of this response, they will in all probability modify their behavior and exercise their innate prudence. With this development the question of abortion for the unwed will become a moot point.

Nature does not act capriciously. When it comes to love, a most powerful life force, neither should men and women.

If Tom Edison did not eliminate those experiments which were non-productive, we would still have gas lamps on Main St.

If humans do not eliminate from their behavior those actions which create and perpetuate alienation and frustration, they will never attain peace in their lives nor permit it to develop in others.

Positive social changes will occur when women use their sexual ability with intelligence and faith in themselves and the Creator of life. Man can do nothing to improve the state of the world without woman's genius.

12. PEACE IS A PAIR OF DOVES, UNFETTERED

Once, years ago, this writer saw an exquisite Oriental rug for sale. Noticing my interest, the dealer asked if I detected anything unusual about it. When I confessed that I saw nothing out of the ordinary, he asked, "Do you see the birds?"

Immediately up from the rug arose innumerable birds - pink birds with yellow wings, blue birds with green wings, gray birds with ruby wings. They all but twittered!

Tucked among the curlicues, leaves and flowers were birds so cleverly designed that they were hidden from view until the means for detecting them was provided. The words of the dealer added not a stitch to the rug. The birds were there all the time, but assistance was needed in order to see them.

It is the same difficulty which prevents people from achieving interpersonal harmony. The means has always existed, but couples have lacked the necessary clues. Without clues to the appropriate behavior, they are unable to achieve their full potential and so peace eludes them.

Let it be recognized that there will be no peace between nations, races, nor the haves and the have-nots until it exists first between husband and wife. If man does not act like a love-filled being outside the home (events in Iran, Afghanistan, and El Salvador come to mind) it is because man has not been a love-filled being inside his home. International agreements and Congressional legislation are futile if spouses fail in their commitment to one another.

And coitus every night of the week and twice on Sunday is not synonymous with fulfillment. As Rollo May stated, "Sex for so many people is an empty, mechanical and vacuous experience."

What has robbed sex of its dynamism? It is man's failure to realize that childbirth is as much a part of the marital encounter as is coitus. Because of his ignorance, man has created a corporeal communication gap which prevents married couples from attaining the level of development that is their due.

Contrary to popular belief, in his preoccupation with sex a man is not seeking pleasure. Rather he is responding to a stimulus that drives him to search for psychic/spiritual health which is as strong and as deep within him as is his will for physical survival.

It is not the unicorn that man pursues but rather union. As in the medieval tale of that elusive creature, it is only through the good graces of a gentle maiden that such a goal can be achieved.

In our culture this impetus for genuine fulfillment is thwarted by our technological approach to childbirth. Instead of a husband receiving his wife's genital gift in a meaningful manner, this presentation is made by her to a stranger, to whom she owes nothing.

A husband ends up cheated and disappointed when his wife hands herself over to the medical specialists. She, too, suffers because of her action. Each and every Adam is entitled to get his rib back. Eve must realize that birth is her opportunity to return Adam's rib. Then no longer beholden to him she will be free to take her rightful place at his side and no separation, no division will exist between them.

Lovers should retreat to the dimly-lit seclusion of their bed-chamber for this ultimate in sexual encounters. There, as the wife releases into the eager hands of her husband that babe which they together created, he will cup his hands into a receiving organ permitting him at last to step up to that long sought-after higher level of existence, "fully human, fully intelligent, and free," to use the words of Dobzhansky.

This life-changing event, never to be forgotten, will be indelibly recorded on his brain. Wilder Penfield, M.D., director of the Montreal Neurological Institute of McGill University, wrote, "What the brain is allowed to record, how and when it is conditioned - these things prepare it for great achievement, or limit it to mediocrity." The age of mediocrity is past if man will but submit to the sensory stimulation of love's complete act.

The separation of lovers during the experience of birth has arrested the biological development of man upon which psychic and spiritual growth is contingent. Man culturally cut off from a maturing experience remains imprisoned in a lower state of existence, allowed to become bigger and older but denied the opportunity for further neurological and physical development.

Not so those who have fought to become fully human. Like the butterfly which is free of the laws governing the cocoon from whence it had emerged, truly human spouses will discover new conditions exist because of their new consciousness.

According to Abraham Maslow the psychology that we now teach is based upon the study of "crippled, immature, and unhealthy specimens." As psychological functioning and physiological functioning are not two separate orders of phenomena, but rather two aspects of an interacting unit, Maslow's cripple-psychology cannot manifest itself other than in the cripple-physiology which is what we have today. With couples behaving in a different manner during the experience of birth, however, present limitations will cease to exist.

Marriage is a pledge of life-long intimacy. When brave, young lovers use the birth experience as a vehicle of marital intimacy, an exquisite something will be released from the warp and woof of the human fabric and a new world brought into being.

Prisoner of Love

God is not dead
but lies trapped in creation.

Come, Woman,
treasure of the universe!
Strike thy flint
and bring forth Limbo's prisoner -
the <u>Easter light</u>!

M. Moran

PART THREE

For Those Who Intend to <u>Really</u> "Go All The Way"

13. LOVE TALK

It is not necessary to try to become an instant-obstetrician by mastering medical (or midwife) texts in order to give birth in a fully humanized manner. Childbirth is a normal, womanly, physiological function. What's more, it is a genital expression, and if a man and wife approach birth as a love encounter, in the same manner as they approached that other genital expression nine months earlier, then their baby will be born quite effectively. And the event will bring greater satisfaction to the new mother and dad than they had ever known.

In the hospital, many of the efforts made to assist the laboring woman are highly technical and require skillful management. This is not so for the woman giving birth at home with her loving husband as her partner, provided, of course, her prenatal care indicates everything is normal. Conditions such as toxemia and diabetes are serious. They are the exception rather than the rule, however.

Those details which are of great interest to an obstetrician are of little concern to a homebirth couple. It is unnecessary for a couple to concentrate on them and to do so may even be found to be a distraction from the experience of birth.

Does the nursing mother worry about the color of her milk, its composition, or the number of ounces a baby gets at a feeding? No. She just relaxes, tucks her infant close to her with her nipple in his mouth and he gets his belly filled and thrives beautifully. The foregoing are some of the details the formula manufacturers must be concerned with, however, in order to produce an acceptable substitute which can nourish a baby satisfactorily.

Does the loving couple give any thought to the texture or color of the woman's cervix, or to the pH of her vaginal mucus, in order to make a baby? No. They just snuggle close and "do what comes naturally" and the next thing they know – Momma's pregnant! These are details that an obstetrician must give attention to, however, in order to artificially inseminate a woman.

Similarly, the birthing couple need not give a thought to the length of the contractions nor to the length of the interval between them. Neither is it necessary for man and wife to know how many centimeters the cervix has dilated. Just to insert her finger tips into the birth canal and to feel the top of the baby's head is enough reassurance for the mother. She then knows that her baby is there and advancing. And this sensation invariably causes her to instantly relax her legs and pelvic floor, which aids in the descent of the child.

In the hospital, technologists have worked out a certain routine which is effective in getting a child to be born. At home, loving couples have worked out an entirely different routine which is just as effective and, incidentally, is a lot more fun!

As the moment of birth approaches, one's husband should not try to be a pseudo-obstetrician. He is a loving spouse and it is in this role that he has his expertise (or should!)

Love is a dialogue and marital love is a corporeal dialogue, that is, a dialogue of flesh. The vehicle for communicating marital love is touch, of an intimate nature. Therefore, for man and wife to highly refine their tactile communication is the very best preparation for the love encounter of birth.

This requires much patience, care and thoughtful

preparation. During the nine months of pregnancy both should take advantage of their opportunities to communicate marital love and to <u>really</u> get to know each other.

It takes a mother up to 24 months of patience and encouragement to understand and to communicate with her infant. Communication between man and wife takes time and energy, too.

So, young lovers, don't rush through your lovemaking. Those sweet-talking fingers are saying something of great importance. They are saying, "If you love me, you'll show me!"

A woman's ultimate response to her man comes during the birth embrace when into his eager hands her body yields her gift of love communicating, "This is how much I love you."

> "with this ring I thee wed; with this gold and silver I thee give; with my body I thee worship; and with all my worldly goods I thee endow."   –1549 English prayer book

MARILYN A. MORAN

14. PREPARATIONS

There are a few things that must be considered in order to insure a problem-free homebirth. First of all, the mother should be well-nourished. Of course, this is equally true whether she is going to deliver in the hospital or at home. But at home, where there is no spare blood available, it is imperative that conditions such as anemia be avoided by good nutrition.

Mother-to-be, and father-to-be, should be careful to get adequate protein, to eat as many fresh fruits and vegetables (especially green vegetables) as possible, and to stay away from highly-processed 'junk' foods, which are only empty calories with little nutritional value.

The pregnant woman should also be cautious about taking medicines. Even the popular, over-the counter drugs such as aspirin and sleeping powders alter the mother's normal physiology and can adversely affect her developing unborn baby.

Cigarette smoking is also unwise. A pregnant woman who smokes two packs a day blocks off the equivalent of 40% of the oxygen supply to the fetus. The incidence of stillbirths, spontaneous abortion, and low weight babies is considerably greater for smoking mothers than for non-smokers.

Alcoholic beverages should be avoided, too, for they also can negatively affect the developing child.

It is very important that the pregnant woman get adequate prenatal care. A good doctor can determine many important things about the baby, such as its position and the placement of the placenta. Toxemia, anemia, and diabetes, which can complicate pregnancy and birth, are all detectable through prenatal care. So, find an understanding doctor or a good midwife. Ask questions and get your questions answered. If your doctor has a reputation for turning away homebirth couples you may have to keep your plans from him. (But when he finds out after the birth, maybe he will think twice about turning down the next couple.) Doctors have been educated at great public expense and they do have a responsibility to serve the needs of the public.

According to an article in *Family Practice News* (March 1, 1978, p. 49), "Homebirth is just as safe as hospital delivery for low risk mothers." You have a right to know whether you are a low risk or high risk candidate and the best way to find out is from a specialist.

> Caution: Don't get an X-ray unless it is <u>absolutely</u> necessary. God never intended that the developing child be exposed to such a powerful force. It would seem prudent to avoid sonograms for the same reason.

As the day of birth approaches a few specific preparations should be made in anticipation of the event. A clean, comfortable area should be selected for the place of birth. This could be the couple's bed, a bean bag chair or a reclining chair in their living room. It could even be the floor in front of the fireplace if that happens to be the mother's favorite spot for relaxing. Whatever the room that is selected, it should be one that can be kept warm easily, if necessary.

It would be well to pick a spot not too distant from the bathroom as mother will have to make frequent trips to relieve her bladder and bowels. For her to have to climb a flight of stairs to get to the bathroom during the late stages of labor would be a nuisance.

A path of newspapers from the selected birth area to the bathroom would prevent the carpet from getting soiled, and is easily removed afterward. So, have a stack of clean newspapers set aside for this purpose.

Also, it is possible that although a certain spot may be picked out ahead of time for the birth, mother may feel more comfortable somewhere else at the last moment. Therefore, be flexible at all times.

If a bed is selected for the place to give birth, make it up with fresh linen. Be sure to have a sheet of plastic under the mattress pad to protect the mattress in the coming weeks. Some women have such a good milk supply that they leak during the night during the first week or two following birth. Later their supply regulates itself to the baby's demands, and this is not such a problem.

After the bed is made with clean linen, then the whole bed should be covered with another large piece of plastic. This can be a painter's drop cloth from the hardware store, a plastic table cloth, or even an old (clean) shower curtain. If none of these are available, a heavy layer of clean newspapers would do.

On top of all this is placed a sterilized contour sheet, to securely hold everything in place. It is on top of this sterilized sheet that mother will give birth. Afterward, it is a simple matter for her husband to peel off the sheet and the protective layer just beneath (be it plastic or newspaper) revealing the freshly-made bed all ready for mother and baby to enjoy.

Although babies are born in many parts of the world without the benefit of ultra-clean surroundings, it is important to make an effort to provide as germ-free an environment as possible for birth. In addition to safeguarding the health of the baby, it will help prevent the mother from getting childbed fever, which took the lives of many women years ago, when the importance of cleanliness was not realized.

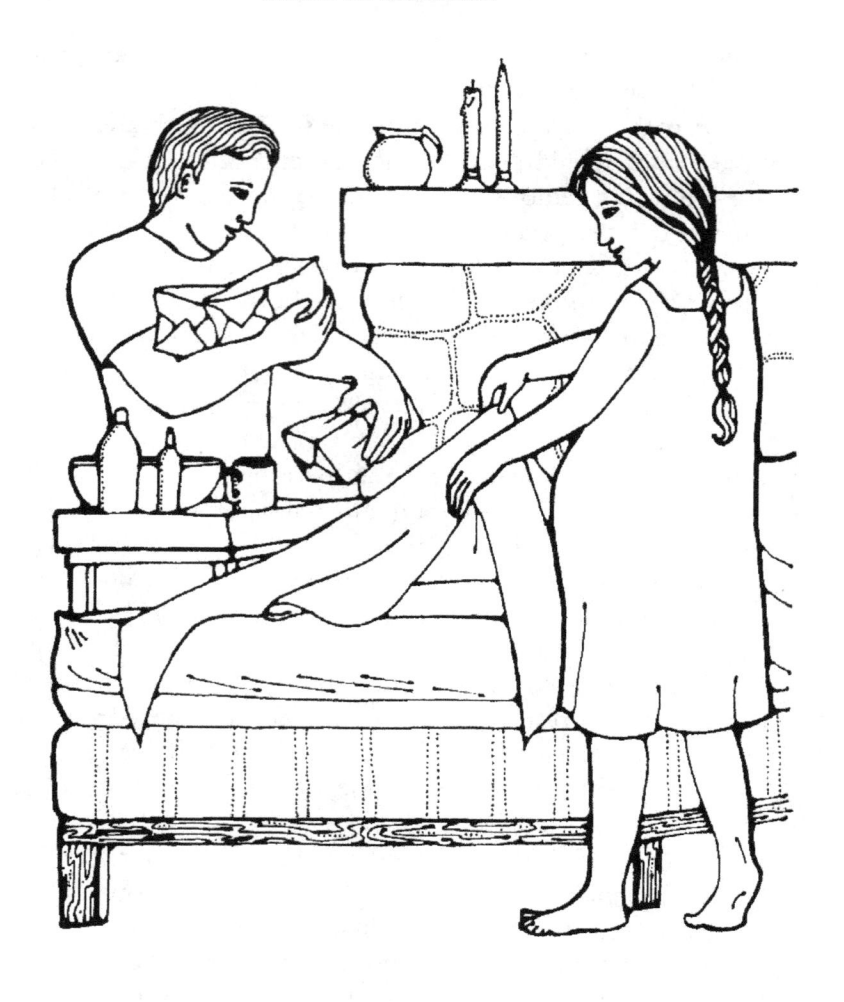

At home, there are none of the super-germs floating around that are found in most hospitals. Nevertheless, there are germs. An effective provision for maintaining cleanliness for the baby's benefit and for mother's, too, is as follows:

1. A dozen or more soft, absorbent rags (old towels, Children's tattered pajamas, sweatshirts, etc.) should be washed, bleached and dried either in the sunshine or in a clothes dryer.
2. Fold the rags and wrap them together, 4 or 5 at a time, in neat bundles in brown paper and tie them with string or seal with masking tape.
3. Place the bundles in a preheated oven at 325.° Put a shallow pan of water on the bottom shelf of the oven. This will help prevent the rags from getting scorched. Roll a potato into the oven, also. When the potato is baked, 1¼ - 1½ hours later, the rags are completely sterilized.
4. Stack the cooled, sealed bundles on a table close to the selected area for birthing. The above should be done about a week before the baby is due. If the baby should be late, just repeat Steps 3 and 4 every week or so.

The bundles will be opened as needed, and a couple of rags placed under mother late in labor as birth becomes imminent. When the cloths become soiled or wet from amniotic fluid, they are whisked away and fresh ones substituted.

One mother did not prepare her sterilized material until the day her baby was born. She reported that the warm rags felt very soothing to her 'bottom.' So, it might be a good idea to rewarm the bundles in a slow oven (200°) during the early stage of labor.

An old midwife device that homebirth couples are finding convenient is the newspaper pan. This is a large, flat object, made of newspaper, with a rolled rim about 2 inches high. As birth becomes imminent a few of the sterilized cloths are spread in the 'pan,' and it is then slipped under mother's bottom. The advantage of the newspaper pan over manufactured bed pads is that the rim prevents the amniotic fluid from splashing across the bed and down on the floor.

The newspaper pan also makes an excellent receptacle for catching the expelled placenta. It is preferable to a large pot or bowl, as recommended in many books, as it does not have a cold, hard rim which could be uncomfortable under mother, especially if the placenta doesn't deliver for 30 minutes or more.

To make a newspaper pan:

1) Stack 15-20 sheets of clean newspaper, unfolded and fanned around on top of one another to form a circle.

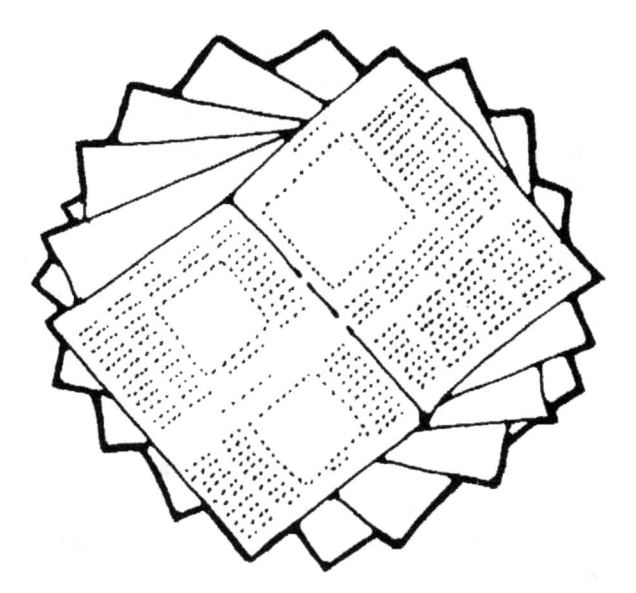

2) Then roll up a rim all the way around just as tightly as possible.

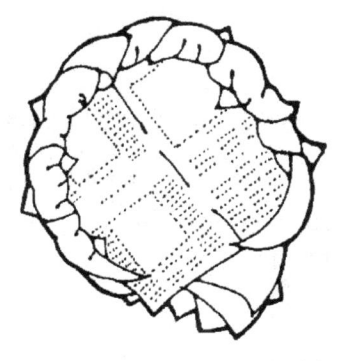

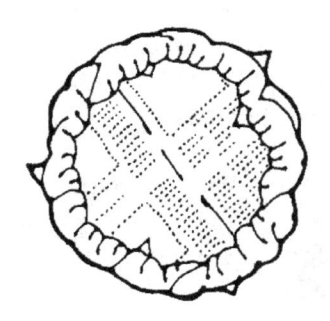

If the rim will not hold its shape satisfactorily, it can be reinforced in this manner. Take a large plastic trash can bag (the size that fits a 30-gallon can) and slit it along the folded edges. Then trim each corner so that they are curved slightly. You now have two pieces of plastic, measuring about 30"x 37." Fold over a one-inch hem and stitch on the sewing machine all the way around each piece of plastic. Insert a string in this casing and tighten slightly. You now have what looks like two giant shower caps. Rest a newspaper pan in each, rim side up, pulling the string until the plastic fits the pan snugly. Tie a knot in the string. You now have

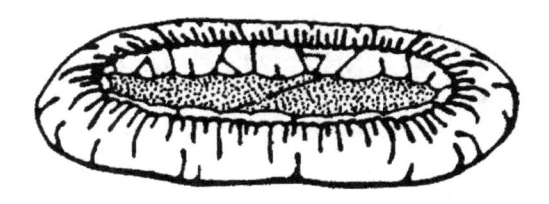

two newspaper pans that will maintain their shape, are easy to handle, and are super waterproof.

Three of four newspaper pans should be made and stored near the area selected for birth.

When the bundles of sterilized cloths and the newspaper pans have been made, the expecting couple usually gets a very good feeling about giving birth at home. Now that they have prepared their 'nest' for the newborn, Mother and

Dad invariably look forward to the event with even greater eagerness than before.

A few more preparations should be taken care of first, however. The following is a list of items to gather together for the birth:

Betadine soap (or some other antiseptic solution, such as Zephiran chloride, properly diluted according to directions) for father to scrub his hands and arms with, up to the elbows, prior to the birth. His finger nails should be cleaned and trimmed, too.

Mother should shower early in labor, and then cleanse her hands and genital area with the antiseptic solution, also.

White infant shoe laces for tying the cord. Make sure only white ones are used. Infant shoe strings are narrow and easily tied into a tight, square knot around the cord. In case you have forgotten, a square knot is made according to the formula, "left over right and right over left." The shoe strings should be boiled for 10 minutes in a covered pan, ironed dry, and carefully placed in a new plastic bag until needed. Or, after being boiled, they could be covered with alcohol (along with the scissors, see below) if they are not boiled until the day of birth.

Scissors for cutting the cord. These also should be boiled for 10 minutes. Then drain off the water and pour in rubbing alcohol to cover them. This will keep them sterile, and prevent them from getting rusty, which is what would happen if they were left in the water.

Rubbing alcohol

Infant ear syringe to suction mucous from the baby's mouth and nose to clear its air passages. Some texts say not to boil the ear syringe as the rubber will lose its tone. If it is new, however, one 10-minute boiling should not harm it.

Olive oil. It is an old midwife technique to massage the mother's perineum with olive oil to promote elasticity of the tissues. The bottle of oil could be placed in a bowl of warm water first, to take the chill off. Also, it is a good idea to transfer the oil to a carefully cleaned, plastic squeeze bottle. In that dispenser it is easier to apply the oil just where it is needed.

<u>Box of Kleenex</u>

<u>Extra towels</u>

<u>Heating pad</u> - for mother if she feels a chill. If she doesn't need it, a receiving blanket could be wrapped around the heating pad, so as to have a nice warm blanket in which to wrap the infant the moment he is born.

<u>Ice chips</u> - to relieve mother's thirst while in labor. Weak tea tastes good, too.

<u>Bundle of infant clothes</u> - including diapers and diaper pins. Also, have several receiving blankets available. Newborns have a way of soiling everything when they soil their diapers.

<u>Clean change of clothes for mother</u> - plus hospital-sized sanitary napkins and belt.

<u>Unsweetened grape juice</u> - for mother to drink afterward. It helps to restore the blood which she has lost. She might like some juice during labor, too.

<u>Blanket</u> - to cover mother and baby afterward. Mother's arms are an excellent warmer for baby, but a blanket thrown over both of them (unless it is the middle of summer) will prevent any possible chilling of the infant. Remember, the uterus is 98.6° and room temperature is generally around 70.° That is quite an abrupt change for the baby. Therefore, the child should be covered immediately following birth.

<u>Oral thermometer</u> - for mother to use to check her temperature if, in the days following birth, she doesn't feel too well.

Emergency Childbirth, by Gregory White, M.D. Most homebirth couples like to have a copy of this book on their night-table, for ready reference. It was actually written for firemen and policemen and explains the birth process in simple language.

In addition to getting the above supplies ready for the birth, there are a few other details which should be taken care of, too. Arrangements should be made for the care of the other children in the family if birth should occur during the daytime. According to Margaret Mead, most non-induced births take place at night. There are exceptions to every rule, though, and you just might be one of them!

Even if there are no other children in the family, it is nice to have an extra person or two in the house at the time of birth. There is nothing as distracting for a birthing couple as having the phone ring over and over, and to have no one there to answer it for them. We know of several mothers who, during labor, received long distance phone calls from their own mothers. So, it is well to have someone there to handle Ma Belle, if for no other reason.

If others are invited to help at the birth, they should be in-formed as to what their duties are ahead of time and be given a chance to practice them. For instance, if someone is going to be expected to maintain the supply of ice chips and hot tea, they should find out beforehand how to operate the ice cube tray, and where the tea bags are kept, as well as the honey and lemon. Husband and wife are going to be too involved with each other during the birth to want to run to the kitchen to help out the helper.

An emergency back-up plan should be worked out well before the baby's due date. It is rarely put to use when the mother has had good prenatal care, when she has been careful about her nutrition during pregnancy, and when she and her husband are well-read and confident in themselves and in what they are doing. However, it provides a little 'security blanket' for all concerned and is worth the little time it takes to arrange.

Someone should know the route to the hospital, and also which door to enter late at night. Frequently, the usual doors are locked after hours, so scout out the place ahead of time.

As the due date approaches, make sure there is gas in the car at all times. And Dad, be sure to have someone else to drive it for you.

The doctor's telephone number should be taped to the

wall above the telephone. The number of the hospital should be taped there also. If you should decide to go to the hospital, all you have to do is make the two calls and then be on your way.

Mother should have her blood type card handy.

A word about filming the event - Don't!

Granted, it would be nice to get a picture of your toddler's reaction when she is brought in to meet her new brother or sister. But to have someone present taking snap shots or movies of the birth is to introduce an element which could very easily interfere with the flow of love energy, and produce a negative effect.

What would have happened nine months earlier if a photographer was present when the child was conceived? A photographer cannot add one iota to your experience; he can only detract from it. Because a woman gives birth so rarely, nothing should be allowed to mute the experience for her or her spouse.

15. FOR HUSBANDS ONLY

Your role is to support and reassure your wife as she gives birth to your child. She can do it. All she needs is your encouragement and the security of knowing you care.

There is one simple, reliable sign by which you may judge your wife's ability to give birth and which should be reassuring to you, too. Nature has provided every mother with the ability to nurse her baby. The breasts start to change and develop shortly after conception occurs. If mother-to-be has noticed a change in her breasts (or you do) you can be certain that her uterus, pelvis, and birth canal have changed too, in preparation for pregnancy and birth. This is because the hormones which are responsible for breast development also work on the other reproductive organs at the same time. Sex hormones are not discriminatory. They work on all the reproductive organs simultaneously. So, if change and development is noticeable in one area, you can be certain that the appropriate changes are also taking place elsewhere.

Therefore, during birth your task is not to do anything, except be a loving husband. Nature has done all the rest for you. As one doctor reportedly tells the husband who is assisting his wife to give birth, as he (the doctor) stands by watching, "Don't try to take the baby. Let her give it to you. Let her put it in your hands."

If mother is in a vertical position, i.e., sitting, standing, squatting, etc., she'll do that very nicely, provided she is getting 'good strokes' from you.

The complementarity of man and wife extends right through the birth experience. Each is just what the other needs.

As for practical suggestions on how to get your wife in the mood for giving birth, it would be well to start by stroking her hair, rubbing the back of her neck, brushing her ear lobes with your thumbs, rubbing noses with her, 'necking,' etc. - you should know all the gentling techniques if you have been making the most of your lovemaking opportunities the last several months. Now is the time to put them to use!

Rub her back firmly, up and down, and her shoulder blades, too, always being tuned in to her responses to your touch. Pay attention to all her messages at this time, verbal as well as non-verbal.

Don't rush anything. Proceed slowly as you advance to the rib cage and then to more intimate areas of her body. (She may want you to massage her inner thighs, too.) This is the advantage of do-it-yourself homebirth. Without anyone watching, it is easy to really 'get into' the birth experience, provided all inhibiting factors are eliminated beforehand.

The following is an excerpt of what Scarlett Hart wrote in THE NEW NATIVITY, a newsletter for do-it-yourself homebirth couples:

> ...all I could do was tell Bob how much I loved him and how good it felt as he barely touched me with his fingertips. I had gone to bed nude so rubbing and loving was unobstructed...Just how he managed to support my weight and rub my legs and back, do the perineal rub (sheer ecstasy at this point) and check my progress, I'll never know...If only I could somehow recapture and put on this paper the intensity of the love that I felt for the man who was helping my child to be born. No father should ever

allow any other man to stand in for him at birth any more than he would call in a stunt-man double to take his place during conception. Every nerve of my body was completely bare to be stimulated and all the stimulations were pleasant.

The perineal massage, to which Scarlett refers, is a midwife technique which has been adopted by homebirth couples and is so effective in keeping mother's perineum soft and elastic that even 10-pound babies have been delivered without injury to the mother's birth canal.

As the baby's head becomes barely visible (or sooner, if you prefer) pour some olive oil on the area immediately surrounding the birth canal and just inside, and gently massage it into the flesh. This lubricates the canal and keeps blood flowing through the area, encouraging the elasticity of the flesh. It also has a very relaxing effect upon mother, especially if you have been smooching, rubbing noses and doing other super-nice things together.

As more of the head becomes visible, continue to anoint the area, gently stroking down one side of the opening and up the other, back and forth, using two fingers.

When a plum-sized portion of the baby's head is visible, apply counter-pressure to the surrounding area to slow down the descent of the baby. One nurse-midwife who had been a missioner in Pakistan for many years said the best way to support the perineal area is as follows:

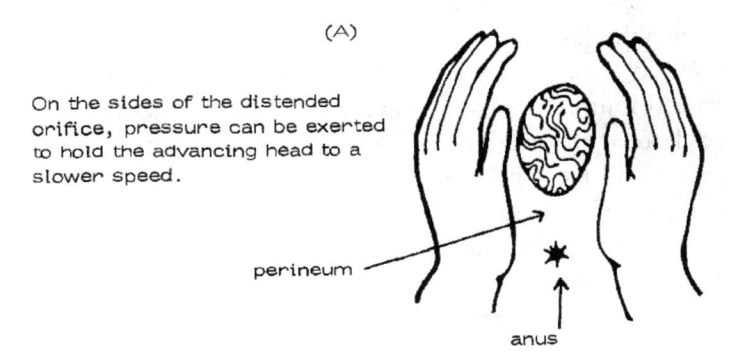

(A)

On the sides of the distended orifice, pressure can be exerted to hold the advancing head to a slower speed.

perineum

anus

If there is a sign of excessive thinning of the perineum as the head advances (indicated by the perineum turning white) then a little downward easing on the sides can loosen and relieve this tension.

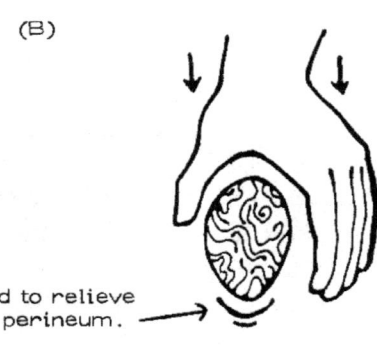

(B)

This area will be loosened to relieve tension at the apex of the perineum.

The other hand should be on the head to control its speed a little.

One mother said she wanted to touch her baby's head as it started to emerge so she supported the top of the birth canal with her hand (as in Fig. B) while her husband supported her perineum from below. She said the sensation felt very good, and she never tore.

Incidentally, a doctor who has been doing homebirths for many years said that even with perineal massage a tear will occur in about 50% of the cases. The midwives at the Stephen Gaskin Farm report similar results. However, on the Farm it is the midwives who always catch the baby. It is never the father who does it.

When a father catches his own baby the likelihood of perineal injury occurring is greatly reduced. According to a newsletter of the Wichita, Kansas, chapter of the Association for Childbirth at Home, Int., which contained a survey of various aspects of births in the area, "The ACHI home birth mothers whose husbands catch have a 12% rate of tears."

This illustrates the exquisite complimentarity between man and wife. Nobody is better able to assist a woman in childbirth than her own husband.

When birth is experienced as a husband/wife love encounter, the problem of so-called 'sensory overload' is non-existent. On the contrary, it is sensory deprivation that women have suffered from all these centuries. In the arms of you, her loving spouse, your wife will get all her needs met, beautifully. Have no fear!

As for what you should say to your wife to help her open up and release your baby into your hands, there is probably no better phrase to use than the one she says to you when you are presenting her with your gift of love. You'll know, and she'll know, the right thing to do and the right thing to say as you bring the dialogue of love to completion in the birth embrace.

God has the birth interaction all planned out for you. All you have to do is to cooperate with His divine plan, and enjoy it!

If you are tempted to call upon Him for guidance at any time, don't hesitate to do so. Remember what He said, "Whenever two or three are gathered together in my name, I am with them also."

16. TEN USEFUL SUGGESTIONS FOR THE LOVING BIRTHING COUPLE

1) As most non-induced births occur at night, remember to rest every day as the due date approaches. You don't want to go into labor when you are overtired.

2) In the early part of labor continue normal activities. Walking is beneficial. So is gardening together and then showering. Prior to all the important events in life (Baptism, Holy Communion, Bar Mitzvah, your first date, etc.), great care is given to washing and dressing the body. This is one of those times! Prepare for this significant 'rite of passage' with care and ceremony, dressing in the special garments which have been selected for the event. One mother we know made and embroidered a special shirt for her husband to wear. Why not make a matching shortie gown, Mother, for yourself? (Even though you may not have it on long!)

3) Put to use those favorite massage techniques that you have worked out together the past several months. And, Mother, don't forget to give your darling husband his share of tender attention. You are not the only one that is expecting, you know.

4) Guard your privacy.

5) Turn on your favorite music and dance, or just sway to its tempo. Walking around is beneficial during labor, so waltzing around is probably even better.

6) Smile encouragingly at each other, and lightly stroke each other's cheek, and around the mouth. And don't forget to kiss!

7) Welcome each contraction and yield to it. Don't brace yourself. There's no need to run away from the sensations of birth. Perineal massage will help encourage relaxation and the descent of the baby, especially if it has been practiced during pregnancy. In *"Sex During Pregnancy,"* (Redbook, Nov. 1977) Elisabeth Bing and Libby Colman suggest lovemaking as a suitable activity for couples during the early stages of labor. They go on to say, "Stimulation of the breasts and other erogenous zones releases hormones that seem to pick up the pace of labor." Without any third-party watching them, a husband and wife can really get into the experience of birth, and breast stimulation will not just "seem" to pick up the pace of labor, but will definitely assist in the happy culmination of the birth event.

8) As the moment of birth approaches, mother will find it reassuring and helpful to put her finger into the birth canal and touch her baby's head.

9) Mother should be vertical for giving birth (i.e., sitting, squatting, or standing). Did you know that men's arms are longer than women's? Maybe God planned it that way so a husband could cradle his wife in his left arm as he supported her perineum and the baby's head with his right hand.

10) If mother feels a burning sensation during the birth, she should pant like a dog. This will prevent her from pushing, and will give her perineum a few more moments to slowly yield to her infant's head. Also, mother should not push until the urge to do so is overpowering, and she just cannot do otherwise.

One final reminder - Don't forget to kiss!

17. CARE OF MOTHER AND BABY

When the baby is born one of the parents' first concerns is to make sure she is breathing. Generally all that is necessary is to carefully lift her up and place her face down on mother's abdomen where both Mother and Dad can stroke her back. As a rule this is all that is necessary to stimulate the baby to take her first breath. If there is some fluid in her mouth it can dribble out if you lower her head a bit. Sometimes the baby will let out a little cry. Rarely does the child cry very loud and long.

Sometimes there is some mucous in the child's nose or mouth which can interfere with breathing. This can be removed by compressing the bulb of the rubber ear syringe and carefully inserting the tip into the baby's mouth or nostril to extract the mucous as the bulb is released. If the baby is crying the air passages are clear and suctioning with the syringe is not usually necessary.

(For further instructions concerning this subject, read *Emergency Childbirth*, by Gregory White, M. D. Two other good sources of information are the *H.O.M.E.* manual (Home Oriented Maternity Experience) and *Spiritual Midwifery*, by Ina May Gaskin. They also are available from the Birth & Life Bookstore, the address of which is in the Appendix.)

As stated earlier, it is important to keep the baby warm. Chilling can cause the child to develop respiratory trouble.

An excellent warmer is mother's arms.

Within minutes the baby could be put to the breast, if she is interested.

It is not necessary to tie and cut the cord right away. Usually couples wait until the cord has stopped pulsating, which may be 20-30 minutes after the birth. Then Dad can tie one shoelace on the cord about one inch from the baby's body and the other one about two inches further away. After that the cord is cut, with the sterile scissors, between the two shoestring knots.

In the meantime mother has probably passed the placenta. If not, be patient. It will probably come in an hour or so. There should be no bleeding during this time. Again, refer to *Emergency Childbirth*, the H.O.M.E. manual, or *Spiritual Midwifery* for more detailed instructions.

Mother should be kept comfortably warm and given some grape juice to drink. Then she should be given whatever she wants to eat. Don't be surprised if she is real hungry.

She should be assisted to the toilet, and she may want to take a shower, provided she doesn't feel faint. Otherwise, a sponge bath, in bed, would be adequate until later.

There is no need to make phone calls to relatives and friends right away. Mother and Dad should take time to enjoy their new little one and revel in the thought of what they had experienced together. These are precious moments. Make the most of them. They can't be repeated in a hurry, as you know.

Even in the days following birth the new father should be permitted to spend plenty of time with his wife and baby. He should not have to go to work for several days, nor should he be expected to go out shopping, etc. He, too, has gone through an important "passage" which requires time for its completion.

As for circumcision, if your baby is a boy, read up on the subject ahead of time. Many couples today decide against having it done, once they have done some research about it.

In order to avoid childbed fever, Mother should be very careful about her personal hygiene for several days following birth. Her sanitary napkins should be changed frequently and each time after emptying her bladder she should pour about a pint of warm water over her genital area to cleanse it, and wipe with tissue from front to back.

If her temperature should rise a few days after she gives birth and she feels ill she should be seen by a doctor, midwife, or Visiting Nurse, without delay.

The answer to any question a new mother might have about breastfeeding will be found in the La Leche League manual, *The Womanly Art of Breastfeeding*.

18. PERFECTION

If you look around, you can't help but be amazed at the exquisite provisions nature has made for the maintenance of life on this old planet. The sun comes up each morning right on time, and each Spring the robins return from the south without fail, as the crocuses appear, poking up through the melting snow. Nature, or God, has certainly done a magnificent job of designing this world of ours.

But most women are less than excited about nature's plan for birthing human babies. They'll tell you, "It hurts!," implying that God made a mistake when it comes to women giving birth. God made no mistake, however. It is we humans who have made several mistakes in our customary management of childbirth. One of the biggest mistakes is for a woman to automatically turn away from her husband at the moment of birth.

At the midwives' conference in El Paso, one midwife spoke about how she feels when she determines that labor is not progressing normally and she decides to take the woman to the hospital, and turn her over to an obstetrician for a C-section. Regretfully accepting her limitations (in not having become an OB herself), she confessed, "I'm frustrated as hell when I can't follow through."

Her frustration is nothing compared to that of a husband who initiates a love dialogue and then, because of groundless fears and cultural taboos, he is prevented from following through with the interaction. In the end he is like one standing in front of a two-way mirror, knowing his loved one is on the other side gesturing to him, but being unable to see her.

Well, many women today are breaking through the obstructing barrier. They want their men to have access to them, and it is well that they should. For women have as much to gain as men by interacting. Among social beings it is the only way to maintain peace and harmony.

So, young lovers, don't hold back, but yield to the mystical force of marital love in all its manifestations at the moment of birth, and you will discover how faultlessly the human body works. God planned it that way for you. You will see. He doesn't make mistakes.

PART FOUR

Personal Accounts of Homebirths

THE BIRTH OF REBECCA LYNN CRANDALL
November 5, 1971

My husband Leslie and I will celebrate our 10th wedding anniversary this year. Our fourth child (and third daughter) is now four months old. What follows is the details of the pregnancy and birth of each of our children. The first three were born in the hospital. The youngest was born at home.

We wanted a family from the start but it was two years before I became pregnant. We were both terribly excited and I rushed off to a doctor at the first thought of my being pregnant.

From my little worldly experience that was the only thing I knew to do. A doctor was considered like a god and no one else was capable of delivering a child. Of the mysteries of birth I knew little, nor inquired much.

My doctor, a general practitioner, was the family doctor of a good friend who had given birth to five sons. She had complete faith in his method of putting one under for the whole ordeal. Tiny spider webs of doubt crept into my mind, but these were pushed aside by the modern habit of reporting, "My doctor said such and such..."

The pregnancy went well. I had no morning sickness. I swelled up fast and very much enjoyed being pregnant, jokes and all. The baby was due in late September but the month passed on and still no baby arrived. There was also no change on my part about being 'put under.' After all, it was the expected thing - ether and trialene shots, I believe they were called.

Labor started early on a Wednesday morning. It was very slight labor but as it was my first baby I didn't know this. The doctor admitted me to the hospital and here I was to stay until Friday, when my baby was born, or extracted, to be more accurate.

It is all a blurred memory now. It was pretty blurry even during the days after the birth. Endless hours of walking up and down corridors; nurses saying "Try harder;" the doctor giving anal exams and when I cried I was told, "You are not having a baby. You *are* the baby" - It was nightmarish. Leslie was left to sit in a waiting room through all this.

Finally, I delivered on Friday, October 18th at 10:30 PM. I awoke the next morning exhausted and lonesome and hardly aware that I was a mother. The baby was a husky, lusty 9 lb., 6 oz. boy.

It was unthinkable that I would do anything but breastfeed. The five children in my family were nursed and the five in Leslie's family were also. I intended to continue the tradition. The nurses were not very helpful, though, and tried to discourage me.

The hospital stay was fun, however. I ran around (despite 18 stitches in one spot and 10 in another) and adored the babies and had delightful company in my 4-bed room. It never occurred to me that my delivery was anything but routine, and I was all set to get pregnant soon and have a little sister for Wayne Allen.

I nursed Wayne six months, but fed baby food from the first weeks and gave him juice, water, and milk from a cup. He weaned himself to a cup and was eating completely from the table. I felt this was very 'cute' and encouraged it. He was very chubby, and weighed 30 pounds before he was a year old. But, I never was close to him. At seven years he is a slow learner in school with a gross motor control problem, which is usually outgrown by age nine. I have since learned that this is a common condition of a baby born after a long labor and when over-exposed to drugs.

When Wayne was eight months old I became pregnant for the second time. It was another easy pregnancy, with no morning sickness and I didn't get so big and heavy.

Labor started around 6 AM on March 6th. I was fully prepared for another three day ordeal and so was the doctor. I was sixteen days overdue this time. We went to the hospital around 8 AM and by noon the doctor came to check on me.

The nurses, I felt, ignored me and indicated that I was wasting space there. It seemed like days that I was left alone in that dingy labor room. I had declined the offer of all medication, not because I wasn't planning to have it. I just felt if I was going to be hours in labor I didn't want to be doped all that time.

Around half past three I began to feel differently. But, when I told the nurse she said my mind was in more of a hurry than my body. Fortunately, a pleasant, concerned, dedicated young nurse came along and sure enough, it was only minutes before the baby was to be born! What scurrying! It almost made me laugh. I couldn't believe I was in labor. This wasn't my idea of the 'pain' of which I had always heard.

The doctor was located as I was being wheeled into the delivery room and just inside the door I gave birth to my darling daughter, Christina Robin, who weighed 6 pounds, 15 ounces. It was then that I got my first frightening glimpse of the delivery room with its bright lights and tools.

I had managed to give birth without a drop of medication. It was one of those accidental deliveries I had heard about. It was not so bad. It was wonderful, really.

I was an old hand this time at nursing and didn't let any nurses 'bully' me. Also, I enjoyed the thrill of saying I'd come successfully through an unmedicated delivery, which was almost unthinkable to the other women, some of whom were having their 6th and 8th children.

There weren't plans for another baby soon, but I did get pregnant again not long afterward and nursed Robin only the six months I had nursed Wayne. When I was eight months pregnant and Robin was 11 months old she came down with spinal meningitis and a brain infection associated with it. She was hospitalized for three weeks and almost didn't make it in the first days. The day she came home my parents came from Pennsylvania to live with us for a while.

A few days later I went to my doctor. I had chosen a young doctor in a different town and was planning to go to the newly-built hospital there.

This time I was prepared for labor and delivery. I had read many books from the Hatch Library in Vermont and had faithfully carried out a combination of Grantly Dick-Read and Lamaze exercises. I learned in those few months that having a baby wasn't a secret or ritualistic thing. I had become acquainted with a young woman in Massachusetts and through our correspondence we discovered together that birth was a natural experience and something to be enjoyed rather than to be dreaded.

It was agreed that Leslie could be in the labor room and in the delivery room also for this birth. This was something we were greatly looking forward to.

At that visit to my doctor, just after Robin came home from the hospital, it was discovered that I had infectious hepatitis and a bad kidney infection. Into the hospital I went for three weeks, during one of which I was in isolation. I was lucky to have my mother home with my family.

I wasn't due for two weeks after I got out and fully expected to be late by several weeks again. Around 11 o'clock on April 10th, Easter Sunday morning, my labor started. I didn't tell anyone because I didn't want to miss out on my ham for Easter dinner. After dinner I knew that I had to head for the hospital, ten miles away.

I was excited and looking forward to having this baby. I got in the hospital and was 'prepped,' when it was decided that I should go right into the delivery room. Again, I was just inside the door when baby Hope Leslie arrived - and

Leslie missed it. While he was scrubbing and gowning he stopped for a smoke. He got to the door and was told the good news.

I was wheeled right back to my room, and my baby was wheeled the other way. This tore my heart. I wanted her with me.

I called my Mom, who was just washing up the dinner dishes. She really didn't believe that I had time to get to the hospital, much less have the baby. Leslie took the phone and convinced her that she was indeed a Grandma again.

I was very much bored with the hospital this time, perhaps because I had spent so much time in and around one the past month. I missed the two children at home. I hardly felt I knew Robin and now to come home with a new baby would be even harder on her. It all worked out all right in the end, but we decided we would not have any more children. I nursed Hope for only six months, and she was my first child to have a bottle, which was my mistake for letting someone give her a bottle while I was busy.

Three years later we were both thinking in terms of another child, but I couldn't seem to get pregnant this time. We applied for foster children and sure enough, as soon as we were processed I found myself pregnant and was very much elated about it.

It was another easy pregnancy. In the years since Hope was born, I decided I would have my next baby at home. My dear friend in Massachusetts had had her son Matthew at home the year before. Therefore, I knew it could be done.

I had joked while pregnant with Hope that I would have her at home. Afterwards, I resolved, "My next will be born at home. I'm not leaving the kids." Also, we had moved into the new home we were building, which was ideal for a do-it-yourself homebirth.

I couldn't wait to tell my mother my plans. I was sure she'd share my enthusiasm, but she did not. Even though she had three of the five of us at home, and me without a doctor, she was very much against it. So, I did not mention it to her or anyone but two good friends. I just let my family think I would go to the hospital.

I had another doctor this time, an old friend of my husband. He was the plant doctor at his mill and was only four miles away from our home. He was a very modern, free-thinking man, but I never could bring myself to tell him of our plans for fear he would react as Mom had.

During the last few months of my pregnancy I read *Emergency Childbirth* and *Commonsense Childbirth*. I also had a chance to read a collection of homebirth stories, and I exchanged letters with some of the women who had had do-it-yourself home births. They gave me much courage to go on with my plan.

Carrie, my friend in Massachusetts, had many helpful hints about things that she had found to work well in their home birth. Leslie was a great help, too. He was quite confident that we would have an easy time. He is not a reading man and although I read parts of various books to him I always wanted him to read ALL I had. He never did. He just felt birth was a very natural occurrence and it would go off the way the Lord always intended it to. This gave great strength to me. He never doubted for one minute but what we should stay in our own home for this baby.

A couple of weeks before the birth one of my so-called friends went to my doctor and told him what I was planning. Although the doctor never let on he knew, he tried to scare me with a story of high blood pressure. I had not gained a lot of weight and I was feeling excellent so I didn't really concern myself as much as he would have liked me to. (It came out at my six-weeks check-up that this was all a hoax to scare me into the hospital.) He even talked of putting me in the hospital and inducing labor. I was on the verge of not returning for my check-ups, I was so upset.

He was very kind about all this, I might add. I'm not in the least against doctors, just some of their ideas. I hate to see them thinking that they are indispensable regarding childbirth.

Finally, November 5th, I woke up with labor pains. I

was very happy about it. I knew it was THE day. Leslie decided to go to work, and I was to call him at the first sign of strengthening pains. I spent the day walking around hoping the contractions would get stronger. But they just kept steady, about every ten minutes apart, all day long.

Early in the afternoon I got out the sheets I had sterilized. I made up our bed with a rubber sheet over the mattress, followed by a clean sheet, a plastic table cloth, and a drawsheet. I had folded a clean sheet at the bottom of the bed in case I got cold. I wanted to make things as easy as possible for Leslie since he would be doing much of this work.

I had received a large floral diaper bag as a shower gift and in here were the baby's clothes and sterile sanitary napkins and the things I'd gathered together. There were boiled and wrapped scissors and shoelaces, gauze pads, peroxide, alcohol, and Q-tips. I didn't get fanatical about a lot of stuff. I just had on hand what I had read that others had used.

I sent the two older children off to school, and Hope and I spent the afternoon reading and chatting. My sister called and we talked for nearly an hour without her the wiser that I was in labor.

It was pleasing me that I had so successfully not told the world - I'm a person who has a hard time not blurting everything to everyone. Sometimes I felt very dishonest about it, but in my mind was my Mom's reaction. I had told my brother and he was in complete agreement and couldn't understand our mother's attitude. I can see now it was just motherly instinct, and had I carried the subject on she would have agreed with me.

Leslie came from work at 3:30 expecting labor to have stopped and was surprised that I was still going. I fixed the family their favorite supper of eggs and sausage and pancakes. I was hungry myself. I had bypassed food all day, except for a little chicken soup broth. I knew I was prone to throw up in transition and I didn't want a full tummy (other than the baby)!

Leslie made a joke of feeding me two link sausages, and then labor stopped. He said, "There, it was just hunger pangs." - but bang! Labor was back and in full swing this time. I had long hard contractions about every four minutes.

This scared Leslie and he abruptly said, "I'm going to get Ma." He has never been on close terms with his mother and hadn't seen her in many months. So this surprised me.

I told him to be sure to let her know what she was getting into, with us staying home for the birth. I really didn't like the idea of anyone else being here, but he thought someone should be with the older kids.

His Mom left a company supper to come home with him and was cheerfully ready to just 'be here.'

I didn't let on to them that labor was as hard as it was. I sat in my rocker pretending to be watching TV and doing my breathing. Around 9 o'clock I got the kids off to bed and for a change "Daddy" tucked them in and gave drinks while I just rocked.

Around 10 o'clock I decided I had to be moving around so I begged off tired and went up to our room, just praying that Leslie would follow me up. Finally I had to call him to come up and even then he didn't realize it was 'time.'

He said, when I asked him to stay with me, that it wouldn't be very nice to leave his mother sitting alone. Then the tears came and I told him to leave then. I'd have my baby alone. Then he knew, and stood gently rocking me in his arms for what seemed like the longest time, but it really couldn't have been too long.

I had that feeling of wanting to stand and sit at the same time, and then the millionth urge to go to the bathroom. Of all times, Leslie decided to start reading *Emergency Childbirth*, which laid on the dresser!

It said not to let a woman in labor go to the bathroom. He made me lie down, although I was resisting all along. Then I knew I'd have to lie down, as I felt sick. Up came the soup and the sausage and I started to have the urge to push.

I was propped up with a pile of pillows, and was pulling my knees, while panting during contractions. It was all working very well, but I think too fast for Leslie to get his mind on. He said he saw a bit of blood and I panicked for a small minute. Then he told me to relax. The manual said that it was to be expected.

He grinned and said, "Mama, it won't be long. I see some hair." During that contraction and the next one I panted, so as not to tear.

Out the baby sweetly slipped with a cry before she was all the way out. This cry brought Irene, his Mom, tearing up the stairs. She simply thought labor had stopped and that I had gone to bed, so she was mightily surprised.

His mother was great. She just took charge and knew what to do. After having five sons at home, and three of them <u>alone</u>, and having assisted at several other deliveries, she knew what was expected and began the clean up.

The afterbirth came with the next contraction following the baby. This surprised us all. We put it in a large baby bath tub for the doctor to examine. That is, if he would come.

Rebecca was so fat and clean and beautiful. She had gobs of long black hair and looked so different from my three bald babies. I put her to nurse right away, but she was not interested. So, I just held her, checking toes and fingers and chubby limbs, while the others cleared things up.

Then Leslie decided to tie the cord. It looked for all the world like the dull gray, loopy electrical wire I had been chiding him to practice on. He decided he didn't like my shoelaces so he got some nylon cord and he put it and the scissors in the dish of alcohol. He tied the cord in two places, really longer than I felt necessary but at this time I wasn't about to discourage <u>his</u> part in the miracle. He had difficulty cutting the cord and said he was tempted to get his trusty jackknife out.

He took and weighed the baby. She was right around nine pounds on our rickety old scales. He remembered the camera and took two pictures of her. Then he went to put the after-birth in the cold cellar and the sheets to soak.

I put Rebecca back to nurse. This time she nursed right along and fell asleep there.

Irene put her in the little bassinet which we had ready and I got up to change and to use the bathroom. It seemed so good to be home and to peek in on my sleeping children. I climbed back into bed to hold and admire the baby and Irene and Leslie decided to go have coffee and to bring me some milk and toast with grape jelly.

A little later as I was completely relaxed but too elated to sleep Robin peeked around our door and said, "I heard a noise and it went 'Waaa-Waaa.' Do you know what it was?"

I motioned for her to come, and Hope was right behind her.

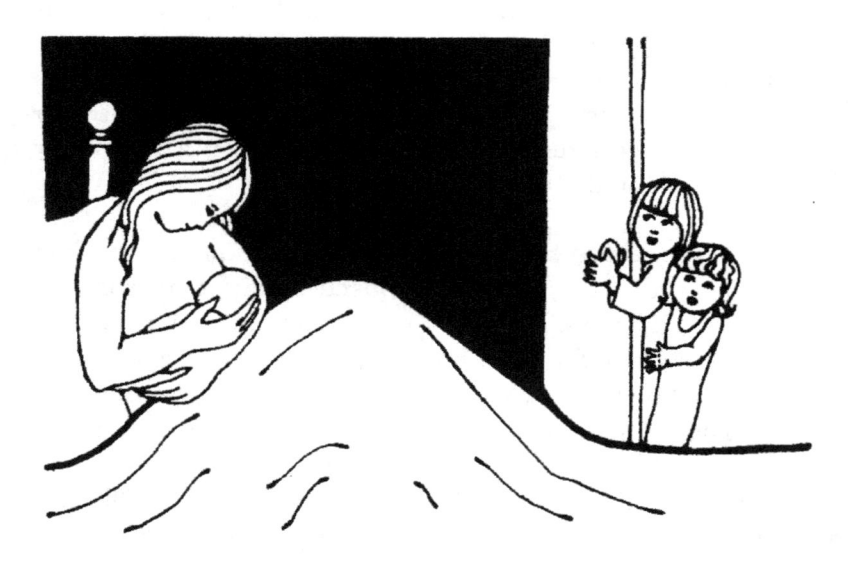

They were so excited to see the baby; they didn't want to go back to bed.

Leslie came to bed shortly afterward. We put the sleeping baby in her bed and tried to go to sleep ourselves, without much success.

The doctor was called the next morning and he came around at noon. We didn't know at the time that it wasn't any surprise to him. He said everything was fine. Yes, the cord was tied a little long but he was sure Les was proud of it, so he left it as it was. He came back three times to see us. He sent the visiting nurses out also, and they were so interested and proud of me. I felt like quite a grand person to hear them talk. Never once did they talk down to me as some nurses are apt to do to a younger person. They even asked <u>me</u> question after question!

A wonderful friend whom I hadn't told I was staying home was thrilled to hear the news and came over with a chicken dinner for us. My family came by and even my mother had to admit she wished she had been the one to be here.

By Sunday night Leslie and Irene finally agreed to let me come downstairs and I got stern lectures from Leslie that I wasn't allowed to run up and down as I was accustomed to. I felt great and by Tuesday Irene went home and I was back on my feet caring for my family and new daughter.

Rebecca is four months old now and weighs 16½ pounds. She is just taking breast milk, and we are hopeful to continue her on just the breast for at least six months and nursing her longer if possible. I'm sure it will be a success.

She has kept her dark hair and has dark eyes, in contrast to our three blue-eyed blonds.

We've been asked if we would do it again. Yes, if we have more children we will. We plan not to go on without taking in foster children, however. Providing homes for those who are less fortunate is important to us, also.

Kathie Crandall, Black River, N.Y.

THE BIRTH OF LUIS ANTONIO SAAVEDRA
February 23, 1975

To many people, especially Americans, the mere thought of having a baby at home is dreadful. The typical husband in this culture rushes his wife to the hospital at the first sign of labor. To do anything else would be considered extremely foolish. However, there are a growing number of not-so-typical, planned, natural births which are taking place at home amidst a warm and joyful atmosphere, where the newcomer is welcomed eagerly by both parents and sometimes even by brothers and sisters.

I would like to share my experience with other expectant parents, and to offer suggestions for those who are planning a homebirth. Our baby's birth took place at our home in Wichita, Kansas. My husband, Antonio, was my attendant. Also present was a very close friend who had some medical background, and who was interested in witnessing first-hand a pleasant birth experience, unlike that which she had had with her first child.

If I may include a short summary of my first two births, I may be better understood in regards to some of my personal viewpoint. They are as follows: Our daughter Ximena Melanie was born July 20, 1972 in Oruro, Bolivia. I spent my last month of pregnancy there with Antonio and his family. My labor lasted about $17^{1/2}$ hours, the first 12 hours of it passing almost unnoticed because of the lack of discomfort. Since I did not speak enough Spanish at that time, Antonio was invited to spend the entire course of labor and delivery with me to serve as interpreter.

Although I had thought about natural childbirth rather seriously, I was not sure that I wanted it. How brainwashed I had been!

During the transition part of labor, I was informed that I would receive no medication, because it is reserved for only complicated deliveries. Luckily, I had read Elizabeth Bing's book, *Six Practical Lessons for an Easier Childbirth,* and I had Antonio's support and encouragement. When the time came to deliver, my genital area was thoroughly cleansed, and since I did not have the urge to push, I was instructed to push hard with contractions. Ximena arrived with a loud, healthy cry.

I was so surprised I laughed like a hyena, while Antonio sobbed. It was such a joyful moment!

Because it was not customary, I did not receive the expected prep, enema, drugs, episiotomy and forceps and stitches routine. However, I did tear slightly and was instructed to pour a solution over the area each time I visited the bathroom. Within a week the tear was completely healed.

Tania Maria was born September 13, 1973, in Jasper, Alabama. My pregnancy was completely normal. However, I did not know when to expect her because I had not menstruated after weaning Ximena from the breast. When my family doctor finally told me that labor would begin at any time, I became impatient and took castor oil. Within a few hours strong labor began and my membranes ruptured. My labor lasted only three hours.

I had arranged to have my baby naturally. Prepared childbirth was unheard of at that hospital, so I was scolded each time I semi-sat with pushing contractions. Later I was told I was lucky that I was not strapped onto the delivery table. I did not need an episiotomy.

I regretted two things in particular about that birth:

First, that Antonio was not able to be present at the birth of his second child; second, that I was put through a mild shock when the doctor immediately placed Tania on the resuscitator. It was only a routine hospital procedure, but consequently I was afraid that something was badly wrong with my new baby. I asked three times if she was okay before I heard the reply, "Yes!" Then I thought I was being lied to! Other things I regretted were 1)1 could not be with my little 14 month-old Ximena, 2) Antonio could not hold his new baby girl, and 3) I had no privacy in my room. I was so happy when I went home two days later.

I nursed Tania for seven months. Soon after taking her off the breast I learned that I was expecting my third child. I looked forward to having this baby my own way, and read all that I could find about childbirth. This time there was more available on the subject than before.

I was determined not to repeat my previous experience, and I found that almost everything was going my way. I will admit, however, that Antonio was furious when I told him of my plans to have my baby at home. First of all, my parents would disown me and blame him if something were to go wrong, because he had not taken me to the hospital. Second, midwives were not licensed in the state of Kansas, and no doctor in Wichita would take the 'risks' of a home delivery. I would have to depend on my husband, who had no real medical experience, to 'deliver' our baby. And, if there should indeed be an emergency, how would we cope with it? Somehow, I had the faith and the knowledge that everything would work out perfectly. I strongly felt that God wanted me to depend on Him and to proceed with my plans for a homebirth.

My approximate due date was February 10th. I was under the care of a highly recommended specialist until December, when suddenly I decided that I would be better off not to further inconvenience myself by hiring a babysitter every week and driving to the other side of town to see a doctor on an assembly-line basis. Each visit was about the same. I was told, "Everything looks just fine," and I resented the joke made of my serious talk of homebirth. I was eating very well, providing my body and baby with the necessary nutrients for good health. I knew better than my doctor that I was healthy and had a healthy, active baby.

I was advised by close friends to continue seeing a doctor in case I should have to go to a hospital in an emergency. I refused until I had gone about a week past my due date. Antonio had just been laid off his job and was due for an interview in Houston at his earliest opportunity. I took doses of castor oil, hoping to encourage my labor. When nothing happened, I saw a new doctor. I must say that I have never been more humiliated in all my life. On the other hand, perhaps he had never been more challenged by a patient.

This young doctor, fresh out of medical school, argued with me for 45 minutes over my desire to have a homebirth. He refused to examine me unless I promised to have my baby in the hospital. Although I have a strong conscience, I resorted to situational ethics as I debated whether or not to consent to those conditions. I had argued that to promise such a thing would be lying, yet the doctor insisted. I promised that if he would just examine me, I would never see him again. He left me alone to make up my mind.

When he left the room, I could picture Antonio out in the waiting room with our two daughters ages $1^{1/2}$ and $2^{1/2}$, pacing the floor impatiently, and trying to keep the girls out of mischief. Antonio had driven our whole family across town through a foot of fresh snow, stopping several times to dig us out, in order for me to be examined so that he might know when to go for his job interview. I knew Antonio couldn't put off his interview indefinitely. We had to at least try to find out if our baby showed any signs of getting ready to be born.

When the doctor returned I said, "Okay." Although I never came out and promised anything, it was understood, although I'm sure the doctor knew my intentions! He told me that he would expect me to have the baby in the hospital and would I be sure to get myself there, to which I replied, "I'll do my very best."

The examination revealed nothing new, and I returned home with the fear that the following week the doctor would want to induce labor if it had not started. That evening I took another dose of castor oil. When nothing happened, we were sure the birth would not be for a few more days. So, Antonio went ahead with his plans to fly to Houston. A friend of mine stayed with me while Antonio was gone. He returned the next day with the good news that he had the job.

Incidentally, Antonio returned with a new optimism concerning our plans for a homebirth. At last he gave his wholehearted consent. He had brought back with him a Houston newspaper to show me an article about a woman giving birth inside an ambulance outside of a hospital because a doctor refused to have her accepted. The doctor said that childbirth was not considered an emergency. Finally, Antonio had overcome his reservations!

I must mention that during this pregnancy I had read many personal accounts of homebirths which a friend had mailed to me. I felt quite confident that everything would go perfectly and that Antonio and I were well prepared. I highly recommend the following books for those who are considering homebirth: *Be a Healthy Mother, Have a Healthy Baby; Commonsense Childbirth* by Lester Hazell; also, *Emergency Childbirth* by Gregory White, M.D.

As the days dragged by, I hoped I would not have to keep my next doctor appointment. Antonio kept reminding me that the sooner I had the baby, the sooner we would be able to move and find a place to live in the Houston area. As Monday grew nearer and I feared the induction of labor, I took my last dose of castor oil and prayed that I wouldn't have to be subjected to the hospital routine. So, with a "Que será, será," I hoped for the best and proceeded to take a hot bath and to wash my hair. As before, when Tania was born, I found new energy and sat up watching TV and crocheting. I was aware of mild, regular contractions, but I chose to ignore them for fear that it was only the false labor that I had experienced so often during the last three weeks. In fact, these contractions were milder than the false or warm-up labor. I told myself that they would just go away when I went to bed, but about the time I decided I needed to go to bed, it became evident that I might not get the rest I was hoping for.

Suddenly, I became aware of the discomfort of the contractions as they started to grow stronger. I tried various positions and breathing techniques to relax and to free myself of discomfort, only for my labor to grow progressively stronger. Finally, I had no doubt that the time had arrived, and I informed Antonio that 'something' was happening. He remained unconvinced, sleeping with one eye open, until I began pacing the floor, panting and seeking more comfortable positions.

I put scissors and new white shoelaces on to boil (for cutting and tying the cord) and I called Brenda, a dear friend who supported me and who was to attend the birth. We were having our second blizzard at this time, and the weather bulletins warned motorists not to go out at all. Brenda left for our house almost immediately, for the usual five-minute drive, and arrived only minutes before the baby was born. During the time I waited my labor almost had control of me, although I was convinced that I could handle everything. I began to doubt myself a little ("Who do you think you are kidding? What comfortable position? What breathing techniques?").

I wondered if indeed I could be in transition. My contractions were so close together, I could barely get out a sentence between them. In a rush, Antonio and I prepared our bed and also a low, firm twin bed which, at the last moment, I decided was more comfortable and convenient.

On top of the freshly made bed we placed sterile white sheets and homemade pads to go under my hips. I made frequent trips to the bathroom to urinate, and discovered that the only way for me to get relief from my contractions was to assume a semi-reclining position with my knees spread apart. During the last trip to the bathroom I decided to cleanse myself thoroughly since we did not know how soon birth might be. While I was soaping myself I felt the bag of water protruding. I then wasted no time in assuming my birth position on the low bed, with my back to the wall. I was semi-sitting with my knees bent and was propped by my arms behind me. In this position pressure was taken off my lower spine during contractions.

Brenda arrived and sat nearby to keep me company. She brought her blood pressure equipment and made herself useful, besides giving me emotional support.

I found it easier to relax during the long, hard contractions if I closed my eyes and concentrated on relaxing, resting my chin on my chest, mouth hanging open - as suggested in Sheila Kitzinger's book, *The Experience of Childbirth* - and breathing as deeply and as rapidly as I felt I needed to. I concentrated on relaxing and found that by doing so, I could blot out pain and that I could feel myself progressing. I knew it would soon be over. However, I had to concentrate intensely on relaxing in order to remain in control.

My water broke and sent a splash across the room all over the newspapers which had been placed on the floor only moments before. I felt an urge to push during a couple of contractions. Then, as the baby crowned, I relaxed as I felt the stretching of the perineum. The uterus gently pushed out the baby's head. Immediately, he took his first breath and his body turned all by itself. Then, the rest slipped out and our baby gave a healthy little cry. He was placed on my abdomen and Antonio announced excitedly, "It's a boy!"

I immediately put the baby to my breast and nursed him. He didn't waste a second. I don't know how to describe how wonderful it was to hold the warm, slippery, squirming new life that God had brought into the world.

The light in the room was not very bright, though not dim. Luis Antonio was wide awake, looking around at the overhead light, at his father, and at me as I nursed him.

I drank a big glass of orange juice minutes later. I felt cleansed, as one often does after physical exertion. And I felt happy, at peace, and prayerful with reverence for the great miracle of birth which had just taken place. I felt fulfilled as I observed the joy of Antonio, at the birth of our first son. We were humble, yet proud.

All we could do for 15 minutes afterwards was talk unbelievably about everything that had just happened. I continued to nurse Luis until the placenta was born. To our surprise, there was no big gush of blood at this time. Antonio, Brenda, and I examined the placenta, which appeared intact, and then it was wrapped in newspapers and disposed of. About 20 minutes had gone by when the cord was cut. By that time the cord was completely thinned and white, with no more blood for the baby.

Antonio tied two sterile (boiled) shoelaces near the navel, about an inch apart, then carefully cut the cord with our boiled scissors. It was very simple and clean. There was no blood in the cord.

Luis was placed on the baby scale which we had borrowed, and weighed in at 8 pounds, 6 ounces - my largest baby. We did not wash or wipe off any of the protective vernix, the heavy white cream which coated his skin, concentrated in all the wrinkles. In two days there was no visible vernix remaining. We washed only his diaper area with clear water. Two days after Luis was born, when it was possible to drive through the snow, our pediatrician came to the house and examined our perfect baby. It is rare to find a doctor who makes house calls; this was an exception, because I had talked to him a month before my due date and explained our plans for the homebirth. Influenza was epidemic at this time, so the doctor agreed that a house call was safer than bringing the baby to his office.

Since we did not wish to have our son circumcised, our doctor answered our questions concerning care of the penis. Although this subject is discussed in baby care books, there is disagreement among physicians in regard to the best method. For example, one book I have read instructed the mother to push back the foreskin daily to 'stretch' it and to clean the head of the penis. I was under the impression that an uncircumcised baby boy would require special attention or he would encounter problems of hygiene, and possibly the foreskin would never separate and would remain tight. However, our doctor, who was European, had grown up in a culture which did not circumcise males, so I took his advice and caution as well, which was to simply leave it alone. It does not require special care. In fact, problems often develop when the foreskin is forced back too early, causing irritation and sometimes introducing infection.

A few days later, Antonio and I took Luis to the local health department and completed birth registration forms. We ordered certified copies and soon received them through the mail.

In summary, my labor lasted at least two hours, yet not much longer. The membranes ruptured just before the baby crowned. I gave birth in a semi-sitting position, hands behind me, raising my hips slightly during contractions to ease lower back pain. My legs were completely relaxed. My technique was to remain in control by intense concentration on relaxing. Sheila Kitzinger's theory on relaxing worked in my case, and that is as follows: There seems to be a definite link between the use of the pelvic floor muscles and the use of the mouth and jaw muscles. To illustrate this, contract your pelvic floor muscles and hold; you will notice that your teeth are probably nearly clenched, jaws tense and tight. During the latter stages of labor it is important to relax the pelvic floor so that the birth is easier. Pain causes one to tense. If one is able to relax, pain can be minimized.

When a woman giving birth remains in control of her pain, and relaxes, she has mastered the art of giving birth. To relax the pelvic floor muscles rest chin on chest, let mouth drop open, relaxed. Close the eyes. Take deep breaths as rapidly as you feel comfortable. It is best to practice this technique before labor, to get the hang of it. This technique enabled me to relax and counteract the powerful urge to push as the baby's head emerged. This way my uterus pushed the baby's head out very gently and I did not tear. According to some sources, the woman in labor has a natural holding back reflex which causes her to stop pushing as the baby's head begins to emerge. However, from my own experience, I do not recall this in myself; the urge to push was so great when my second baby was born that I ignored the doctor when he told me to stop pushing. I did not tear, but I did over-stretch at one point. I feel that self-control plays an important part in the art of giving birth. Perhaps the fact that I was having my baby at home without a doctor caused me to take the relaxing techniques more seriously and to do my very best, based on what I had read and discussed with other mothers during my pregnancy. And, consequently, when the time arrived, we were confident, relaxed - at least more than expected - and operating automatically and very efficiently. My storybook-perfect labor and delivery were a result of preparation and faith.

Our homebirth supplies consisted of: The book *Emergency Childbirth*, by Gregory White, M.D., an ear syringe, a nasal aspirator, gauze, adhesive tape, cotton, scissors, new white shoelaces, sterile pads (large enough to go under my hips), sanitary napkins, a trash can, Wet Ones, baby scale, tape measure, and a list of phone numbers in case of emergency. We had ready some soft receiving blankets, disposable diapers, and undershirts. However, all we actually used were the pads, Wet Ones, sanitary napkins, a trash can lined with plastic, a receiving blanket, shoelaces, and scissors. We did not immediately need the diapers and undershirts.

Luis did not have a bit of mucous, so we did not need the syringe or aspirator to suction him. We did not wipe out his mouth. Gregory White advised against this in *Emergency Childbirth*. Unless the baby does not breathe and appears in serious trouble it is not necessary. We did not hold the baby upside down by the ankles. Babies born naturally do not usually have mucous which might require draining, and nature takes care of their blood circulation. Personally, I feel that it is cruel to treat the baby that way. It is becoming more common to place the newborn face down across his mother's abdomen immediately after birth until he starts breathing.

About castor oil - certainly it is not a good idea for pregnant women to take this or any laxative on a whim in hopes of starting labor. In some cases, especially problem pregnancies, perhaps it could cause premature birth. However, according to what a nurse and my doctor told me, castor oil is often prescribed to women whose babies are due or overdue, to start labor. My doctor instructed me as follows: mix two ounces of castor oil and about three ounces of orange juice in a glass; next, add one teaspoon baking soda and stir quickly. When the mixture begins to fizz and foam, drink it immediately as it is quite unpleasant. It's heavy and oily.

I was told that it would not harm my baby and that unless the baby was ready, it would not start labor. By experience, I have found this to be true. I felt it was necessary that I take castor oil in the instances in which I did, but I do not recommend it to anyone who simply is impatient for labor to begin. Since Luis' birth I have learned a more pleasant way of achieving the same results without the unpleasantness of drinking castor oil and without the laxative or purgative effects. Women in Bolivia and other parts of South America drink a tea made of dried parsley, and sweeten it as they would regular tea. This tea is supposed to bring on a sluggish or overdue labor, and also late menstrual periods. A friend of mine who lived in Bolivia and who has tried this with two overdue labors says it works. I think I would certainly prefer the tea to the castor oil 'soda' any day!

If I could change anything about my experience of homebirth, I think I would have recorded it all on tape.

I prefer my home experience to a hospital delivery -

there's just no comparison. I feel that the sharing of the beautiful experience of birth serves to draw a husband and wife closer. In my case, a doctor was not present and I depended fully on my husband. His attitude told me, "Relax, you're in good hands. Everything is going beautifully," and finally, after our grand triumph, "Thank you for trusting me and for depending on me - for allowing me to lead you, step by step, through this ordeal, for I appreciate this wonderful gift." Although Antonio never used those words, his attitude reflected the thought.

Antonio still announces proudly, "I delivered my son!"

Monica Saavedra
Wichita, Kansas

THE BIRTH OF HANNAH SMALLTREE
January 11, 1975

We live and teach at a coeducational Quaker Boarding school. Six students share our home, which made our situation for a home delivery quite unique. The entire school community shared in the pregnancy and birth, through their physical and spiritual support. One of the students, Mark, asked to be present at Hannah's birth. Our friends Kathy and Paul, who helped at many other deliveries, were also present, and helped Richard and me bring Hannah to the light.

I had my first contraction around 11:00 Thursday night, January ninth. Thursday was my due date, but we were almost certain that this was not real labor. My body wasn't ready for it. My cervix was still very thick, and the baby hadn't dropped. Still, the contractions continued. They came every ten to twenty minutes, and some were so strong that I resorted to Lamaze breathing. I did not sleep that night; Richard slept fitfully.

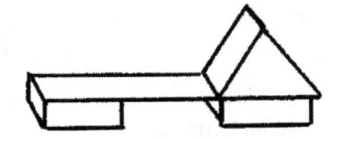

On Friday, we were both tired, but we went about our regular business. I met with the biology class, where we talked about childbirth, and the students listened to the fetal heartbeat. Richard taught his math classes. The contractions continued. We still thought they were false labor, because I had no discharge, no mucus plug, no breaking of waters. Just in case, though, Richard cleaned the room where we planned to deliver, and I checked the bag of supplies we had assembled.

We had decided to have the delivery in our favorite room. It was the room where we kept most of our books, plants, instruments, and records. It was a bright room, and we could keep it warm. Usually the room was furnished with pillows on the floor, but two weeks earlier Richard had built a bed with an adjustable back for the delivery. Now that piece of furniture dominated the room, waiting for the day.

The contractions continued Friday night. I could not sleep; Richard slept for an hour. By one o'clock Saturday morning the contractions were four to five minutes apart. Each contraction used a portion of my energy. I had been having contractions for twenty-six hours and had not slept for forty-two hours. I was already very tired.

Still sure that this must be false labor, I tried to convince Richard not to call Kathy and Paul. I was certain that as soon as we had called them and gotten them out of bed at 2 AM the contractions would stop. I was wrong.

We called Kathy and Paul at quarter to two. Fifteen minutes later I went to the bathroom and found a mucus plug, a small cylinder of mucus less than an inch long. It was heartening to have something happen. At least there was progress.

We put a clean sheet on the delivery bed and I settled down for the serious part of labor. At the beginning of each contraction I would take a deep breath and then start to pant. As the contraction grew stronger I would pant faster, and then slow down as the contraction subsided. I would end with another cleansing breath.

Richard watched me closely and told me to relax any muscles I started to tense. By two-thirty contractions came every two or three minutes, and each lasted about a minute.

I was surprised, and somewhat disappointed, that labor did not take the course the Lamaze books had said it would. Hence, my breathing was radically different from what I had practiced. From early Saturday morning until the moment Hannah was born, I was in the panting, or 'level two' stage. There was just no phase of active labor when I could have used a slower breathing to stay on top. The 'cleansing breath' at the beginning and end of each contraction was essential, as it was my cue to relax completely. Richard would always remind me to take my cleansing breath if I forgot.

By 4 AM my body had used all its reserves. It had been seventy hours since I had slept, and almost as many since I had eaten. At one point when we were alone in the room, I whispered, "I can't go on." My voice was hoarse. Richard offered to take me to the hospital. I was adamant about staying home, however. Whatever kept me going was deeper and more powerful than human will.

Kathy and Paul arrived at four. They brought their new baby, Oliver, who had been born at home just two weeks before. They brought with them an energy and focus that we badly needed. With them, the hardest contractions became the best, because they accomplished the work.

<u>Richard</u>: The room developed a new rhythm which complemented the rhythm of Mary's contractions and panting. On one side of Mary was someone who made hot compresses, and on the other was someone with ice and cold water. As each contraction began, Mary had a hot compress placed on her abdomen. After the contraction ended her face was wiped with a cool cloth, and she was given ice to suck. Others in the room meditated, whispered encouragement, watched for tenseness, panted with Mary, or prayed - anything to send her strength. At regular intervals Mary would get up and walk to the bathroom. She could have used the bedpan, but the walks gave her a change and lifted her spirits. When she left the room the rhythm stopped, like a clock without the pendulum.

When dawn was breaking, the six students who lived with us began to stumble out of bed or come home from morning milking. I scribbled a quick note and asked them to read it to the community at collection. We asked for their thoughts and prayers.

Fatigue was becoming overwhelming as the day progressed. Mary's contractions changed in response to her low energy level. They now came in groups of about five. The first contraction of the group was the strongest; the others became weaker. Then there would be a pause of five to ten minutes. During the pause Mary would go right to sleep. When her body had the strength, another contraction would start and wake her. The rest of us took turns sleeping while the others attended.

All day Saturday labor went on with little obvious progress. It was discouraging. However, the groups of contractions gradually came closer together. By five PM the contractions were almost continuous; as soon as one ended the next began. There was no more rest for Mary.

At six o-clock her waters broke. Now things were happening. You could see that gradually Mary was placing compresses lower. Now they were on her pelvis. The contractions continued without interruption.

By eight PM Mary was feeling the urge to push. Our child was almost ready to leave Mary's womb. The contractions were powerful; this was transition. Mary was using pant-blows now, and blowing continuously when she had to overcome her urge to push. Then there was a pause. With the next contraction Mary had to fight not to push. Finally it was clear that transition was over. Mary was allowed to push. Our daughter was on her way.

<u>Mary</u>: Probably the hardest part of labor was fighting the urge to push. I realized how important it was to wait until I was fully dilated, so as not to tear - but, oh, after 40 plus hours of labor, I dearly wanted my baby to come out. Kim did an internal, and announced that she could feel the baby's head, with no cervix around it. It was TIME!

<u>Richard</u>: Mary held each leg behind the knee, and pushed, each time with a tremendous grunt. First just a

wisp of hair appeared; then it slid back. With each push, a little more of the head appeared. Then it would slide back, but not quite as far. On the outside we were ready. I held compresses to Mary's perineum to help it stretch. Two syringes were ready in case the baby's windpipe was clogged. When the head had almost crowned, Kathy told Mary to stop pushing. Then slowly, like magic, the head came out, followed quickly by the body.

I held our baby. The cord was twice around her neck. We quickly unwrapped it. She blinked, dazzled by the new light, and took her first breath. Mary looked down and cried out, "Richard, she's perfect!"

Mary: I was really surprised at how easy it was to push her out. The students in our house were gathered at the bottom of the stairs at this point. They told me later that when they heard my pushing grunts, they pushed with me, and when they heard me exclaim "she's perfect," they cheered. I don't think I've ever seen anything quite as beautiful as our daughter, purple and shiny, with a head of hair almost as long as her father's, lying there between my legs. Hannah, a new little Capricorn, born one day before the new moon.

Richard: I didn't think much about the blood that followed, but Kathy was concerned. Everyone then became alarmed, except Mary who was radiant and kept insisting that she was fine and there was nothing to worry about. Finally Kathy looked at Mary's color and decided that she couldn't be bleeding that badly and still look so healthy.

However, there was still some concern because Mary's uterus wasn't staying hard. When the cord had stopped pulsing I cut and tied it and put the baby to her mother's breast to see if that would help harden the uterus. She didn't want to suck, so I tried. It didn't seem to help. The uterus would harden up when Kathy massaged it, but it wouldn't stay hard.

The placenta hadn't been delivered yet. Finally, an hour

or so later it was suggested that Mary go into the local hospital. That seemed like a good idea to everyone except Mary who did not want to leave our beautiful baby. She did agree to go, however.

Kathy stayed home with Hannah and her own baby, while Paul and I drove in with Mary.

We arrived at the hospital at one o'clock in the morning (Sunday). There we discovered that our local hospital doesn't expect emergencies at that hour. Everything was locked except an entrance way with a red telephone which presumably connected to someone who summoned the doctors from their beds. However, just after we arrived in the deserted parking lot, another car pulled in. The wife of our family doctor had taken sick, and he had stopped by to pick up some medicine.

He was surprised to see us, but friendly. He unlocked the door and brought us all into the emergency room. After summoning a nurse to get supplies, he checked Mary and declared that she seemed all right. He had her push and the placenta popped out. (I was amazed by how large it was.) He then told us that Mary had a small tear and asked whether we would like it stitched. We decided we would. He did. Then it was all over.

When we got home, Kathy and the two tiny infants, (hers and ours) were asleep on the waterbed. Kathy, Paul and Oliver left. Hannah and Mary and I went to bed. Hannah slept soundly through the night in her cradle by our bed. Mary and I kept waking up to make sure she was still breathing, or just to admire her and remember that it had all happened.

She was so beautiful that neither of us could look at her without crying.

Mary DesRosier and
Richard Kleinschmidt
Rindge, N H.

THE BIRTH OF CHRISTOPHER PAUL DOONEY
August 21, 1969

"Wherever there are two or more gathered in my name, there am I in the midst of them" - and for certain there HE was, in our midst on Thursday, August 21, 1969, guiding Christopher into this world every step of the way!

Labor began at 6:30 AM and the baby arrived that evening at 6:33. The contractions were very mild until about one o'clock. In fact, they were far milder than the many false labor contractions that I had been having for the past three weeks. All day long I was not really certain that this was the 'real McCoy' since I had had no mucus or 'show' to verify true labor. The timing of the contractions was not regular, either.

By four o'clock the contractions were becoming a bit unbearable even though I had no difficulty in relaxing between them. By 5 PM the transition stage had begun and I felt naturally anesthetized. Almost all conversation ceased. It was at this point that Bob predicted that the baby would be born at 6:35 and would be a boy. He was off by only two minutes.

When I had gone to the doctor for a check-up around July 1st, he found that the baby was in breech position. Actually it was not true breech, but transverse (cross-wise). It is a very comfortable way to carry. He stayed in this position until the very final bearing-down sensations started.

When we were fairly certain the birth would take place shortly, my friend Evelyn called another good friend, Terry, who had delivered her own daughter at home six months ago. Terry had to wait until her husband arrived home from work to care for their five children, but she made it here just as I had the first bearing-down contraction. Her timing was perfect.

I had three more bearing-down sensations and the baby was out in sight. Bob guided the head as it came out. It came out with great force and then the shoulders locked in position. It felt to me as though a coat hanger was wedged in the vaginal opening. He turned and then his football player's shoulders came out. The baby cried immediately. As he did so, I could see (perfect view from the mother's angle) a long, stringy piece of mucus just inside his cheek. I put my index finger inside his cheek and simply guided it out. It slid out without any probing or coaxing.

It was amazing to watch his coloring change from grayish-blue to bright red to pretty pink, just as quickly as a traffic light turns from green to amber to red.

We were so fascinated watching his little face changing colors, and clearing the mucus, that I was a bit puzzled since I still had a stretched sensation. His little legs were not yet out! I gave just the slightest push and when they emerged Evelyn said that the cord was entangled around one leg. I slipped one finger under the cord and it slipped off the leg with very little effort, since he was so slippery and wet.

His wet little body turned cold within seconds and he began to shiver, his little lips quivering. So, we left him lying between my knees and put receiving blankets over him, covering all but his chubby little face.

It was then that I noticed two of our children up on the swimming pool ladder, just outside the bedroom window, trying to get a peek at what was going on in the bedroom. They had been in and out of the bedroom all during labor and were all aware of what was taking place. The only view they could get from the top of the ladder was of all our heads hovering over the new baby. When I saw them I waved at them and told them to come on in and see what we had. At first they thought I was just teasing them. They had to be coaxed to call the others and come in. They just couldn't believe that it happened so fast.

It was at this point that we remembered to turn the tape recorder on. Several times during the final stage I had reminded Bob to turn it on, but in all the excitement we completely forgot all about it. However, we did get the baby's second 'song' along with a medley of twelve other voices, all going at once.

All eight of the children had come in to greet brand new Christopher; Rena (twelve years old), Eileen (eleven), Karen (ten), Alan (eight), Nancy (seven), Jeff (five), Jill (two and a half), and Kevin (seventeen months). Then the fun began. All the questions! "Whose baby is it?" "How did he get out?" "Can I pick him up?" We had to remind them that little Christopher was still not disconnected, and they'd have to wait a little while before they could hold him.

When the kids saw Christopher he was not yet a full five minutes old, and they were allowed to stay in the room about a half hour.

I could feel the placenta moving down lower and lower. We moved the baby up onto my abdomen, but the cord was not quite long enough to enable me to nurse him. I had just asked Terry and Evelyn if they thought I could get up onto the bedpan in order to catch the placenta since it is quite awkward to handle, but while they were reaching for the bedpan the placenta slithered out. It was 7:15 PM, just a little over a half hour after the birth.

We had been planning the whole nine months that Evelyn would do all the essentials since Bob wasn't at all anxious to. After reading a collection of personal accounts of home deliveries, I loaned them all to Evelyn to read and she was convinced that Bob would never forgive himself if he didn't at least 'catch' the baby. She has such excellent judgment. Just the afternoon before the baby arrived I told

Bob that Evelyn said she would be glad to come in and help in any way she could, but that she insisted on HIM catching the baby. To be honest, that's all we expected of him. But he ended up really taking over.

The cord had stopped pulsating and was already white, but we waited another few minutes before severing it. We had 1 inch wide twill tapes which had been ironed inside handkerchiefs ready for the tying, but we also had a plastic umbilical clamp standing in the alcohol along with the scissors. We intended to use the clamp and sever the cord in order to remove the placenta. Then we planned to do a neater job later with the tapes but found it unnecessary to use the tapes after all.

We were a bit surprised, in fact shocked, when Bob reached over and plucked the clamp and scissors out of the glass and took care of the cord by himself. He says now the only reason he did it is that we'd never let him live it down if he didn't.

Yes, he did the CATCHING, the CLAMPING, the CUTTING, and the CALLING...calling to brag to everyone who would listen!

On Friday he made eight trips - to the hardware store, the bank, the post office, the grocery store, the tailor, the gas station, etc., and each time when he returned he told me of the people he had told. When I accused him of simply looking for errands to run in order to brag, and said I didn't think there was anyone left to brag to, he said, "All right. I won't say another word to anyone, and if anyone should ask me if I delivered our baby I'll simply say I don't know what they're talking about!"

Right then I remembered an aunt of mine who hadn't been notified the night before. Bob volunteered to call her and he disappeared into the bedroom to make the phone call. Then he stuck his head back out the door again and sheepishly asked, "Is it all right if I tell just one more that I delivered him?"

The baby had black (meconium) bowel movements from immediately after birth up until Monday morning when they began to turn greenish-black. It appears that the extra boost he got from leaving the cord intact until the placenta was born kept him going until my milk came in on Sunday. He nursed for about twenty minutes right after the placenta and he were detached and then later (about 10 PM) for four hours straight! I said, "Boy, would he be in trouble if we were in the hospital, with the nurses warning, 'Only two minutes to each side!'"

I had no soreness or tenderness at any time. After the placenta was delivered I did not bother to massage the uterus the way I have always been ordered to do. I always found that quite painful. I could feel the uterus tightening up on its own. I lost much less blood than I usually do. With my eight hospital deliveries, the doctors have been far too impatient and have always taken the placenta out without waiting for it to come on its own. Evidently the tiny vessels from the wall of the uterus into the placenta had not had the chance to dry up and break away on their own and then hemorrhaged when the placenta was plucked out. This was the first delivery in which I could get up out of bed afterward without feeling the blood gush out of me, and my getting the sensation of blacking out.

I was up out of bed at 8:30 that night to go to the bathroom, and several times during the night. Early the next morning I showered and it felt just great.

I had after-birth pains Friday night, some of them pretty bad. During the day I had some but they were quite mild. On Saturday I walked around the yard, pulled some weeds from a small flower patch, and then bundled up the baby and went next door to visit Evelyn. Saturday night proved to be the worst part of the whole delivery. The after-pains were worse than any labor pains, with the pain shooting right down to my toes. Some women attribute the contracting pains after birth to the baby's nursing. However, my worst ones were at a time when the baby wasn't even nursing, and while he was nursing I had none at all.

Sunday we had Christopher christened while he was still

two days old (five hours less than three days old.) I went to church too and felt just great.

Monday morning his umbilical clamp and stump fell off. I didn't discover until two days after the baby's birth that I had three tears. They were completely painless. Within the week they were healed and the heavy bleeding had ceased within five days.

God has been so good to us. It is my earnest prayer that every mother and father can experience a birth such as Christopher's. You can actually FEEL God's presence. I don't know who the author of this statement is, but I firmly believe it: "Each baby is born with the assurance that God is not yet disgusted with mankind."

This was not just a 'home delivery,' but a SPECIAL DELIVERY, since he was delivered by God himself.

Whenever anyone asks little Jill where we got our baby from she simply replies, "God gave him to us. God lives with us, too."

When one of the other children asked what the vernix was all over his scalp I told them it was to protect the baby's sensitive skin. Jill had her own theory. She said, "No sir. God put that there to make him grow."

Bob and I would be delighted if we could encourage any couples who are anticipating having their baby the natural way, in the natural setting, because we know that without the encouragement of people who have done it we, too, might have missed so much.

Oh yes, about our family doctor. Bob saw him the day after the birth, in the hardware store. When he asked how the family was, Bob told him the good news. He congratulated him and seemed very pleased, and he told Bob not to hesitate to call him if we ran into any complications. We're so glad there's no hard feelings on his part. But actually why should there be? After all, we just got him another prospective patient. Chris, too, will have his share of bumps and bruises, etc., and will need the services of our doctor just as all the rest of us do, in times of sickness and accidents. But golly, gee, who needs a doctor

JUST TO BE BORN???

Marie and Bob Dooney
Lincoln Park, N.J.

BRAD'S BIRTHDAY
August 5, 1979
A Journey Through Countless Galaxies of Experiences All Within the Universe of Love

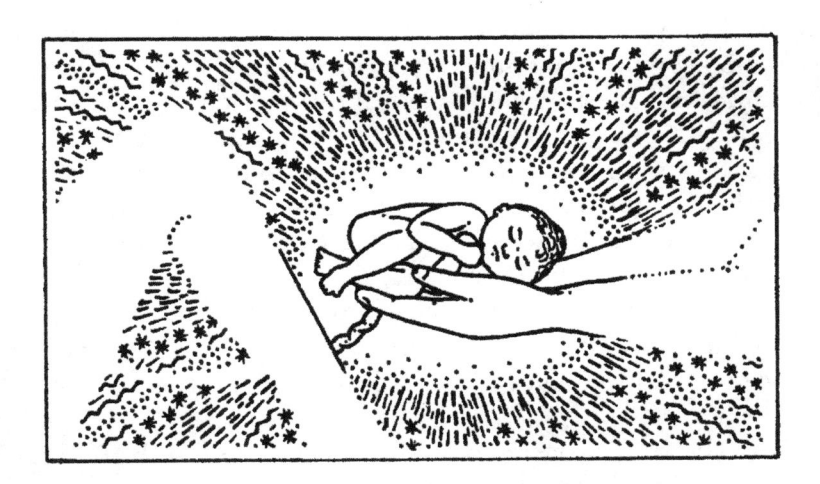

On Friday the third of August I drove over to Poplar Bluff to pick up Bart at work, so we could do some shopping. We ended up buying mostly baby things, final additions to our growing collection. I remember staring at all the ladies pushing shopping carts around with babies in them, and trying to picture myself as one of them. Even at this late date in my pregnancy, that seemed totally unreal!

That night I felt a few cramps. I had felt no Braxton-Hicks contractions during my pregnancy, so I didn't know what to expect at all. I didn't give the cramps much thought, although a couple of times they were strong enough to wake me.

When morning came I was still feeling mild cramps, but I said nothing to Bart and he went on to work as planned. I got up and began skinning and cooking tomatoes for canning. My mother called from St. Louis around noon. I mentioned the mild cramps I felt, and she assured me that I was feeling false labor. She explained that I would feel them on and off for some two weeks or so. That sounded quite plausible to me, as my due date was still about two weeks away.

I went back to my tomatoes. Soon, though, I found that those cramps were getting harder and harder to ignore. So I began timing them, just for the heck of it. To my surprise, I found that although they varied in intensity and duration (5 to 30 seconds long), they were coming very steadily - every 3 or 4 minutes. Was this the real thing? I left my tomatoes and got out a book about birth. From the descriptions I read, my labor sounded half-real and half-false. So, following the book's advice, I filled up the tub. False labor, it said, would be slowed and relieved by a bath, while real labor would continue unchanged.

Once in the tub I reached up and felt myself inside. Something definitely felt different. My cervix seemed much closer, and I thought I felt a hardness behind it - my baby's head?

The cramps were somewhat relieved by my bath. But soon afterward they started right up again, at the same rate but now feeling stronger. Still I tried to convince myself that this was the false labor my mother had spoken of.

Bart got home about 3:30. As I told him of all I had been feeling, I found I had to pause until each cramp passed. With a smile and a hint of excitement in his eyes, Bart suggested I do some walking.

I walked down to the mailbox, picking up the pace when I felt what I finally admitted to be a contraction, not just a cramp. These contractions were beginning to feel quite uncomfortable. They were lasting a bit longer and increasing in strength. It was during this walk that I finally began to accept the fact that the event we had waited so long for was really here.

I got back up to the house and we began some preparations. I did some cleaning while Bart set up the crib. Then Bart got out all the birthing supplies. Quietly I watched him setting things out -was this a dream?

Around 6:30 we ate dinner. I wasn't hungry but I knew I would need the strength, so I ate well.

The contractions were getting so uncomfortable! I went into the bedroom and began experimenting with different positions, trying to find a comfortable way to get through each contraction. Nothing seemed to help! I tried breathing techniques, massages, exercises, - all with very little success. Bart thought I should have been up walking more, but somehow I felt I was past that point. Actually I was torn between wanting to rest and wanting to concentrate and speed up the contractions.

They continued to come at the same rate, but were feeling more and more intense. I could feel the muscles, ones I had never used before, and they seemed to be getting sorer and sorer.

While on my hands and knees, I asked Bart to rub my lower back. Though I was not really having back labor, this felt good for a while. Then I sat upright and Bart continued the massaging, wherever I thought it might help. I stared into his eyes during every contraction and found this helped more than anything. He was trying to time the contractions, but I found it bothered me terribly whenever he'd break eye contact to look at the clock. At one point I felt like throwing that clock away!

It seems I made endless trips to the bathroom. During one I lost my mucus plug. I was glad to see it, for it was my first sign of real progress. Something really was happening!

I never needed an enema, for my body was thorough in cleaning itself out on its own. So much for the nutritious dinner!

Bart helped with towels whenever I needed them. I had

to shed away any impulsive embarrassment, and doing so felt good. Here I was, naked and groaning, sweating and excreting. I felt like I had to strip away layers of cultural 'uptightness,' and each layer shed brought much relief. I began to feel like a confused and frightened animal, hairless and shiny with sweat, yet somehow very close to God.

As the room darkened, I entered the most difficult hours of my labor. I could not seem to direct the energy that I felt ever- increasing in intensity; I was scattered. It seemed I was doing everything all wrong. I was tense and trembling. I found myself dreading each coming contraction. My legs were shaking uncontrollably and I felt awful.

Bart kept telling me to try and relax, and his words echoed endlessly in my mind...I tried! I wanted so much to let go and to accept the sensations, but they were so uncomfortable! We were both becoming disappointed in the way I was handling myself.

Long hours passed and I was still trying to pull myself together, with unbearably little success. It was midnight, contractions were coming every two or three minutes, lasting about 40 seconds. Bart checked my cervix but there was still no sign of dilation. Both of us felt increasing fatigue and some discouragement. Bart complained about the bedsheets falling apart and sliding on the plastic, and I found myself crying, tired and disappointed.

By one o'clock we were both totally exhausted. Suddenly the contractions seemed to slow down. They came far less frequently, every 15 or 20 minutes, and were much less intense. I felt like I had reached some type of plateau, so I suggested we both try and sleep. Bart's eyes, tired and heavy, showed immediate relief at this idea. He lay down beside me, but I was still moaning and panting with each contraction, so he went into the other room to try and rest.

The next couple of hours were by far the worst part of the labor. The plateau was short-lived. The contractions soon began picking right up again. Alone now, I suddenly realized what a difference Bart's presence had made. But I didn't want to wake him. I knew by my own exhaustion how much he needed sleep. He had been sharing each contraction with me and I knew he was as tired as I was. Oh, how I longed to be able to sleep and finish things in the morning!

But contractions came faster and faster, each seeming to reach new peaks of discomfort. I felt an incredible pressure during each one, and this sensation instantly dissolved any concentration on relaxation which I may have tried to muster. At this low point I began to worry that I wouldn't make it through the night. For the first time I began to consider the hospital, only because the thought of a sedative and therefore sleep was such a pleasant idea. I wanted so much to turn off my pulsating body and to sleep!

I had a desperate thought; I would wake Bart and have him check me, and if I had made no progress we would head for the hospital and 'blessed' Demerol. First though, I reached down and checked for myself. Lo and behold, my bag of waters was protruding right out of my cervix! I felt a flood of relief and then renewed excitement...I was making progress!!

I called for Bart, and after quite a while he managed to trudge in wearily and bleary-eyed. Excitedly I told him of the latest development. He looked too exhausted to share my excitement, but stoically he went to the kitchen to make more coffee.

While he was gone, I felt a very strong contraction and the first trace of an urge to push. I pushed just a bit and POP! Amniotic fluid shot nearly five feet, clear over the edge of the bed. Elated, I screamed for Bart. He rushed in, and the excitement returned to his eyes. Surely this baby was really on its way now! It was 3:30 AM, and the fluid was crystal-clear, to our eyes, as healthy-looking as could be.

For me, that great pop! brought sudden and total relief. That unbearable, uncomfortable pressure was totally gone and its disappearance brought me a second wind of wonderfully positive energy. Suddenly I was very, very happy not to be in a hospital!

I wish I could say the whole birthing began at this point, because from here on out it was nothing but beautiful. The contractions were no longer at all uncomfortable. I found I could truly welcome each one as a positive and helpful rush of energy. I sat upright on the bed, against the wall and propped by pillows. Purposefully and peacefully I accepted each contraction as needed help for the work I had to do. Bart's presence doubled the good feelings. He became very beautiful to me. I felt hot during a contraction and chilled in between, so Bart brought me both hot tea and ice water. The contractions came very steadily now, lasting about a minute with two minutes in between.

It no longer bothered me when Bart left the room for coffee or tea or whatever. I felt I both understood and accepted my work. I knew what to do and no longer felt at all lost or confused. Nor was I looking desperately for an answer or solution, either to Bart or to hospitals and sedatives. The answer was within me, the solution was to open up and let it out!

During all these good feelings, I did have a momentary flash of fear. This was when I reached inside and felt something coming...but it didn't feel like a head! It felt soft and rather pointed, like a little shoulder, elbow, or knee. I felt some of the earlier fear and tension beginning to return. My last prenatal visit had been a week earlier, and at that time the head was down but not engaged, being somewhat to one side. And I recalled my mother telling me of my own birth, a complicated shoulder presentation.

I began to feel frightened, but instead of giving in, I called upon God. Surely He had not brought us through such a difficult night into this wonderful state only to let us down! My faith returned and I felt God's presence and I knew all would go well.

Moments later Bart checked me with a flashlight at the height of a contraction. He looked at me and announced in wonder that he saw hair! Lots of hair! Curly and dark - Hair! I was too busy working but I could have cried with joy. I sent a prayer of thanks and felt yet another renewal of positive and holy energy.

Daylight was breaking. Progress still seemed slow, but it was steady and quite definite. As the dim room began to fill with morning light, we both felt we could sense the child's coming presence.

Bart settled himself before me, sitting cross-legged with sterile towels on one side and the flashlight and little dilation chart on the other. He sat so I could rest my feet against his knees and push against him while opening my legs as far as possible. I did this for each of the contractions, which had not changed in frequency but were continually more intense. Bart would massage my thighs, while I concentrated on widening and widening that circle of muscles. I looked at different things while concentrating, at Bart, at the empty baby bed, at pictures on the wall, or just into space at nothing at all.

I had to step up my breathing as the contractions came faster and stronger, and then I found it most exciting to watch Bart's eyes. They would widen at the peak of each contraction - he was seeing more and more of our baby's head!

I kept asking him whether I should be pushing. He'd calmly reply that I'd know when I should, and to wait until I felt I had to. But I wanted the baby born soon!

I was lucky in that I always had time for a short rest between the contractions. I always had a minute or two to lean back and relax totally, to drip ice water across my face and upper body, or to sip tea and stare lovingly and dreamily at Bart, while being careful not to pass out and so miss the beginning of a contraction.

I never went through the dreaded transition stage. I certainly didn't miss it. I had felt more than my share of discomfort earlier in the night. Things just went on smoothly, with no break in the positive feelings we shared. Bart was patient and calm, though I knew underneath he was wishing things would move faster, wishing the baby would come, wishing he could sleep. We talked about wanting all three to cuddle up and go to sleep as soon as the baby was born.

I felt the beginning of an urge to push. I was up to about six or seven centimeters. Bart felt that was not quite wide enough, so I panted through several contractions. The pushing urge was getting stronger and stronger. We found that with Bart helping to stretch me, I was widening to eight or nine centimeters. That sounded wide enough to me. I began pushing, hesitantly at first, then with more and more strength.

I was still sitting up with my feet against Bart's knees. I was busy coordinating my pushes with each contraction, and as I pushed I would lift myself up into a squatting position.

"Is it coming?" I would ask.

"I think so!"

"Farther?" "Yes! A little more each time!"

At the height of each push Bart would lean forward, and as his hands helped stretch me ever so gently, his eyes would widen and widen. The excitement was mounting, the air was charged with energy.

"Come on, baby!" Bart would say. "Come on! Oh, come on. You aren't _that_ big! Come on!" He was nearly choking with emotion.

My feelings were identical, though by now I was hardly speaking, only grunting.

The contractions were coming very close now (no time for clock-watching). I couldn't see the emerging head, but I didn't need to. Bart's eyes were perfect mirrors.

"It looks like such a little head!" he said.

"Good!"

The universe had become the sensation of one big push. The child was inches away from joining us in this world. My heart was pounding. Bart looked electrified. He tried perineal support, but that felt all wrong. This baby wanted <u>out</u>! Massaging and stretching felt best.

Suddenly I felt the most momentous pushing urge of all. I leaned back and lifted myself up and bore down with all my strength (strength that at this point could only be from heaven). I caught a glimpse of a glowing object above his hands, but mostly I remember Bart's incredulous eyes.

"The head!" and then, "Oh, the cord!"

"Around the neck?" I asked.

"Yes!"

"Tight?"

"Yes!"

Not realizing that Bart had already slipped it across the shoulder and loosened it, all I could think was that I had better start pushing, and fast. Without waiting for another contraction, I gave another push, and then whoosh! Our son was in his father's arms, swirling and shining, his rainbow body glowing pink and gray, purple and blue, with spots of yellow and white cream and streaks of green and brown meconium. His "little head" was in reality a Buddha-crown, which topped a chubby face and a plump and lengthy, holy body.

Bart's priceless, passionate words, "Oh God, it's a baby!"

And mine, "A boy!"

He was pretty clogged with mucus, so Bart went to work quickly at suctioning, while I leaned back in ecstasy. He was still quite purple, but I <u>knew</u> he would breathe, for the room was glowing with God's presence. His tight grimace began to relax as he gave a few hesitant and shallow breaths, and as his breathing grew stronger he began to slowly pinken.

He had made it to us! He was here! Alive, beautiful, perfect! Bart and I looked at each other, unbelieving. We were shaken by the miracle, we had been rocketed together into an ecstatic awareness of God's presence and the proof was right here between us: this new being, our son Brad.

I held him while Bart headed for the phone to share the news. I sank back into the pillows, holding Brad's damp little body, feeling totally relaxed and relieved, yet still elated and amazed. I felt like I could have sat there forever, all was perfection and total completion.

I stared into the fresh little eyes and felt a sudden, strong, and deep-seated sense of wonder - for somehow I deeply felt an inexplicable recognition for the child. I felt like I could see an infinite chain of ancestors behind those eyes, and he was the newest link and was right in his place. I recognized him as being just the one I was waiting for, as if I had seen him before and had known him all along.

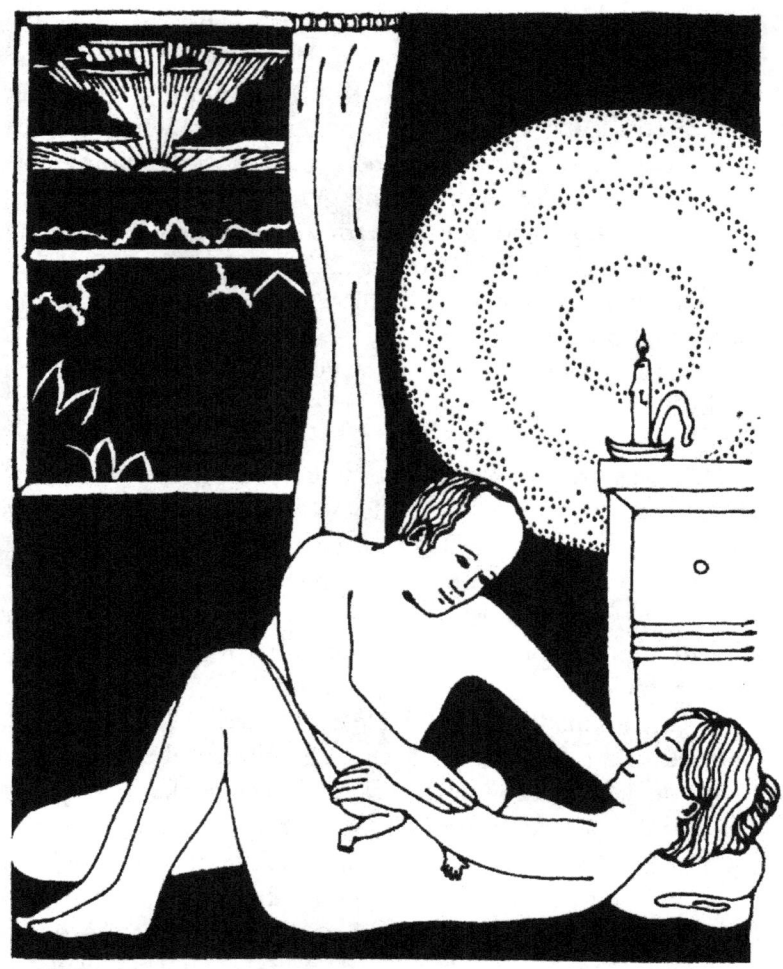

"Oh, of course...it's you!"
Perhaps this is what they call bonding.

BIRTH AND THE DIALOGUE OF LOVE

* * *

This doesn't seem to be a typical love-encounter birthing story. Our experience was one of love, but it encompassed much more. We experienced every facet of our relationship in a deep and rich manner, the negative sides as well as the positive. So we found not only affection and romance, strength, encouragement, and trust, but also fear and anger, discouragement, frustration, and exhaustion. It's as if we delved deeply into ourselves, explored our relationship, and discovered that love means a whole spectrum of feelings and dealings. It was a teaching of the most intense kind, incredible, powerful, and direct, and our gains are immeasurable in all ways but one: the wondrous gift that is our son Brad.

It has been six weeks now since his birth. My strength has long since returned and Brad is thriving. Bart and I are still discovering more and more each day that our postpartum euphoria is here to stay!

Sandy Griffin
Doniphan, MO

The illustrations in this book were done by Sandy.

THE BIRTH OF ANNA MARIE GOODLOE
April 10, 1979
Closeness, and How to Create It

Anna Marie is our eighth baby. Our oldest child is twelve years old. The others were born in the hospital. This child was born at home.

The children were all at home with us during Anna Marie's birth. There were no other adults present. The children were our back-up crew. If we needed hot water or something we just yelled, and they provided it. Otherwise, the door to our room was closed. That is the way we wanted it to be. It was perfect for us. We wanted it to be a twosome, a one-on-one relationship, for the birthing experience. I didn't particularly want the kids there. I get more of their company sometimes than I care to - and at this particular time I didn't want any wonderful questions to answer. I do that all day!

So we thought that we were enough, and it was beautiful because the room felt very full, very contentedly full. There were quite enough people. It was sufficient. For us, two was just exactly the right number of individuals in the room.

I was very slow in the first stage of labor, extremely slow. It never has been any different with all the other seven. It was not any different with number eight. My water broke on Monday at 8 AM. Forty hours later Anna Marie was born. That was Tuesday, at 7 PM.

But it was not intense, continual, un-let-up labor. Contractions were quite sporadic. There was no good timing to them. The books say the contractions go from X number of minutes long, down to X number of minutes, and 'Presto!,' baby arrives. This is not the way I do it. My contractions would fluctuate from an hour apart to two seconds apart, to one good long one lasting several minutes.

During those two days Ken did not leave my side. This was extremely comforting and pleasant for me. Some people are so determined to give birth at home that they would consider themselves to be a failure if they ended up going to the hospital. But when I look back now, had any moment during those 40 hours brought it to an end, every hour had been so beautiful, it was fine. I would not feel like a failure. It was beautiful. Everything up to that point was just great! If by any chance birth just couldn't possibly continue to be at home I still would have felt satisfied with the effort I had put out.

Second stage of labor for me is always extremely fast and it was no exception with this one. I reached transition about 25 minutes til 7. I decided to get in bed. At this moment I became intensely aware of Ken's presence, as if a giant magnet was drawing me in.

The next 25 minutes would prove to be most busy. Though it was proceeding in near silence, it was in reality a beautiful calm. A calm overcast with an absolute clamor of constant and unspoken communication. The quick actions seemed all one fluid motion. It was in this climate of joy, anticipation and keen sense of 'oneness' that Ken's firm but gentle grip on my shoulders helped me onto the bed. As our gaze locked, his soft whispers placed me at the pillows, ready for our greatest moment.

About two pushes delivered the head and two again for the body. So, it was very fast, and it was all over.

I had kind of hoped second stage would be a little slower, so that we'd have more time for smooching, dancing or a few more soft words or something. But there wasn't time for much except for coming up for air. So, that was it. I saw the little head, and then the rest followed. The next thing we knew, Ken was on his knees on the side of the bed. We were all wrapping around, making all kinds of sounds. I couldn't repeat the conversation. I don't know if it made intelligible sense. It was a lot of good noises, anyway.

All I could think of was "Here I am, looking at the most beautiful baby in the world, the daughter of that gorgeous hunk of man at my side, who wore his heart in his eyes and spoke with his hands." How grateful and happy to be me, with him, having her.

The baby made a kind of "M-m-m" sound and immediately went to nursing. That was it. She didn't cry vigorously or get upset or anything like that. The length of the cord surprised us. It was short. In fact baby couldn't get higher than my navel. So nursing was, shall we say, 'awkward,' if not comical. I had to sit Indian-style to accomplish the job. But, we had the will and found the way. Neither of us really minded. We just looked a little different.

The baby weighed 8 pounds, 4 ounces. One week later she weighed 9 pounds, 1 ounce.

We cut the cord a little over an hour after birth because with the children there it was wild, to say the least. Once they appeared it was 'business as usual.' The children had come in very shortly after the birth and the youngest brought her doll and her story book and just camped there. Shortly afterward she was sleeping beside baby sister. There was no problem at all.

Our moments were stolen ones, but beautiful ones, even after the experience. Eye contact alone could say so much. It repeated it all, without saying anything. The dancing, the hugging, the physical contact were fantastic and kissing away had definitely relieved a lot of distress!

Some people might think that they are not prepared enough if they have not had Lamaze or Bradley or any of these things. That's something we have not had, so if you think you have to try three or four methods before you do-it-yourself, it isn't really necessary. As a matter of fact, Ken didn't do a whole lot of reading, either. However, when the day finally arrived he did pick up Gregory White's *Emergency Childbirth* and he read on one page, "be solicitous." So he read, in his best first grade manner, "Are you comfortable? Do you want a drink? Do you need a cover?" - and he went down the list.

Other than that, that was the only reading preparation he did. And I liked it very much, as I was fearful that if he got too hung up on all the books lying around he might be looking into a book and I would rather he was looking in my eyes. I much prefer that 'method.'

I walked and kept in motion constantly right up until the last moment, when it was getting difficult not to push.

I spent a lot of time in the bathroom, also. Ken commented, in fact, that he was wondering if we were moving the birthing room to the bathroom. We had prepared the bedroom, but I was living in there.

After the birth we did run into a complication, postpartum hemorrhage. The placenta took $2^{1/2}$ hours to be expelled, during which time there was quite a lot of bleeding. We immediately started putting pressure on the uterus and this did decrease the blood flow. We continued vigorous massage, up to pain toleration (although it did not cause me any pain or discomfort) and this stopped the flow.

The hemorrhage was an unnerving type of experience, but we had our emergency back-up plan, and if we needed to make a trip to the hospital for blood or a D & C we would do it. But we decided to try A, B, and C first, and if none of the above worked we'd go. The hospital is only eight or ten miles away, and the highways are good.

The placenta hadn't come, and we were tired of waiting. So, after the cord was cut I decided to get up and walk to the bathroom. I had read that sometimes walking around helps the placenta to come. But for me that was a 'No! No!,' for the bleeding increased tremendously.

I had gone only 6-8 feet from the bed when I decided that this was not a good idea, and that I should get back in bed and continue with massaging the abdomen and to be patient. We had newspapers spread out on the carpet like you're supposed to. But, if you are familiar with fresh blood, and how sticky it is - well, it was down both legs, and all over the paper and on my return trip the newspapers were beginning to accumulate on the soles of my feet. As we got closer to the bed we had the Kansas City Star from my thighs down!

In the meantime I had made a little motion with one of my legs hoping to dislodge a few and the cord began to oscillate which, much as a sprinkler system, was getting the walls and curtains. So, Ken had an approximately 45 minute clean-up job that most of you won't experience if your wife stays put!

We got that all done, and really the rest was undramatic. We sat in bed and massaged the uterus, and when I'd get tired or nurse the baby Ken would take over for me beautifully and keep it going. That was the end of the blood flow, and $2^{1/2}$ hours after the birth the first and only contraction came that expelled the placenta, whole and intact, because we checked. And that was it. Everything went right down to normal, as far as any discharge was concerned. In fact it was below par for what I have experienced in hospitals.

We then called relatives and announced what we had done. Their response was SHOCK - period. We had not discussed our plans with them. We didn't wish to argue or worry them if their opinions differed from ours. But they accepted the news quite well, once the horror and the shock wore off to their usual proud grandparent selves.

The baby had no breathing difficulty. She just made little soft noises, like "I'm here. Where are we?" There was no violent crying. Her cord fell off on the fourth day. We were amazed it happened so soon.

At all times I was able to stay completely calm. Throughout the pregnancy as well as the birth I was attentive to what my body was saying and I felt no panic at any time.

Ken took his cues beautifully, from the support, to the massage and everything. It was beautifully timed. We just helped each other, passing back and forth the 4 x 4s or whatever we needed next. We were both in there with it. It was fantastic. He did not need any verbal communication, particularly, for anything, which has to be nature taking its course, as we had to have some good communication system to go on - and that was great.

We found it a very wonderful experience to give birth at home, every bit as wonderful as I thought it would be all seven times - or rather, how I would have liked to have had it. But then, for us perhaps this was just the right time, so appreciated, having waited so long for it.

It was great for us, without having anyone there, as a barrier, or an intruder. It didn't change the way we react to one another. We still communicated, but we did so on a deeper and more intimate level. The words were the same as had been said a thousand times but this time there was another special meaning; it was a little deeper. There was an extra twinkle that you could detect. There were all the warm feelings of, "O dear, you're sweet." Moonlight, soft music and you.

All the magic was working again!

We didn't have much time to ourselves, actually. Fifteen minutes after the birth the doorbell rang. A client was at the door with some papers for Ken. I often wonder what kind of an impression he had, because I think Ken went to the door with some newspapers still stuck to him. ("The last guy didn't pay!") That was one of the fastest checks we ever received.

Anyway, as Ken helped the children to find their pajamas and get ready for bed there was something melting between the walls. You could feel the warmth and the closeness, no matter how many rooms away he was.

And I think that was one of the comments that Ken made, "I feel so close." And that was the way it was. I couldn't have imagined being so close. There wasn't anything to be said. It was all silent, and it said so much.

The message is simple. We've learned that:

We made love and became parents
We had a homebirth and became lovers!

After all, I had come to him as a bride to be fulfilled. To whom else should I turn to be a mother'? How natural!

Ken's comments:

It's hard to explain exactly how you go from "I'd never do it" to "I'd never do it any other way." But that's where I come from. It all seems like a fairy tale that should begin "Once upon a time." Besides, I know we'll "live happily ever after" because the good feelings just linger on and on.

The roles aren't hard to guess. They're very appropriate. It seemed only natural to treat Laura like a queen and it was such a high seeing and holding our little princess. I felt just like a king.

In the beginning my reluctance to have a homebirth was genuine. But by the last months of our pregnancy I was looking forward to it and wanted a home birth myself. What can I say? It was <u>great</u>! I don't regret it!

Laura and Ken Goodloe
Stilwell, KS.

THE BIRTH OF JASMIN LUTZ
August 24, 1978
The Best Way to Have a Baby

After my wife had two very easy but very frustrating hospital births, I finally consented to having our third baby at home. Our original plans were to find a midwife, but being unsuccessful, we decided to 'go it alone.'

We had heard of the Birth At Home League and after taking the classes I had a whole new insight to having a baby at home. The training proved to be valuable beyond price, but the mental attitude of all concerned at the classes was the shot in the arm I needed. Finding all the positive energy instead of the negative vibrations we had been encountering was a blessing.

Where can I start telling of the beautiful birth we had? Or, shall I say 'love encounter.'

When my wife picked me up from work, she told me that "tonight's the night." I believed her because it was her body, and she knew with the others. We had supper, and Moonshadow kept puttering around the kitchen.

She had been having minor rushes through the evening; nothing extreme, just an awareness of a baby wanting to get out. We let our neighbor take our other two children, and were alone.

Moonshadow felt comfortable walking, so several times we went outside. When inside, I was buzzing around with last minute preparations. Our bed had been made a week before, so all I was really doing was killing time.

At about nine o'clock the rushes were getting stronger, so Moonshadow told me to kiss her, and let me tell you - I became really aware! We kissed with each one after that, and I could actually feel the energy that Moonshadow was feeling!

We practiced breast stimulation, and in between rushes sometimes we danced. Moonshadow didn't stay in one position, but moved and changed positions whenever she wanted. We kissed and hugged like we haven't done since we were dating, and I kept assuring her of how well she was doing.

At about 12:10 AM she was experiencing some pretty heavy rushes, and so decided to get on her hands and knees. I was getting pretty excited by now, and when her water broke in a couple of minutes, I was really ready to explode!

Moonshadow decided she would be more comfortable sitting upright against some pillows. Right after she turned over, I got down to see what was happening. I was surprised and thrilled to see the baby's head crowning. I told Moonshadow that I saw the head and she said, "This baby is ready to come out. It wants out," and the next moment the baby's head was out. Not more than one minute later, Moonshadow helped with a little push and the rest of the baby came out into my hands.

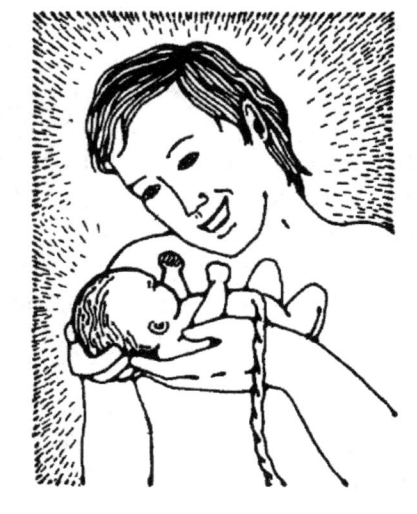

I will never be able to describe the feeling that I experienced as I moved the baby onto my wife's stomach. We were both laughing and crying at the same time. I was so excited that I had wrapped the baby up and had not even noted what sex it was. I peaked under the blanket and laughed and cried, "We have another girl." Our second. Nothing I had ever experienced before, or shall after, will match that feeling that night.

Now, one month later, I still look at my baby girl and know that I am the first person to ever touch her. My wife had given me back the gift of love which I had given her nine months before. Our love has grown even stronger than before, if that is even possible. To me, now, there is no other way to have a baby. I only pray that more people will come to know the joy that I have known by having a homebirth.

His wife's account:

Wednesday, at 4:00 PM, I had a bloody show. I knew we'd have a baby that night. I began having irregular mild rushes at about 5:00. After supper I took a warm bath and lay down for a nap for an hour. Then I got up and made a birthday cake for Aragyn. His birthday was August 25th, and I wanted to make sure he had a cake for it. Still the rushes were mild and irregular.

At nine o'clock labor began in earnest. I remember sitting in our rocking chair riding with an intense rush. With the next rush Aragyn came to me and we kissed. It was so tremendous! Half of the intensity left me and I felt suspended! We were one!

During rushes, while kissing, I kept thinking I was a part of nature, a piece of a natural force such as a storm, wave or flower and needed only to ride with this energetic force. I wanted to calmly let nature work me to bring this child to us and physical contact with Aragyn made this calmness possible.

We danced some. We were always kissing, hugging and touching. When I felt the baby pressing down we lounged on the bed. I felt the pressure one more time. Then my water broke, Aragyn then took his place to catch his gift and with the next rush we were looking at a little grey head! I was so amazed, and knew Aragyn was too, by the brightness in his big blue eyes. With the next rush a baby squirted out of me into Aragyn's hands.

He immediately put this slippery, slimy, little creature on my belly. As I hugged this scrunched-up child we laughed and cried, for there were two small cries and we knew we had a healthy baby. We'd done it! Those moments were so electrifying I can feel the thrill whenever I remember.

About 45 minutes later Aragyn clamped and cut the cord. He took his new daughter and held her close, a joy he'd been denied before.

We were still waiting for the placenta. I had the urge to stand, so I did. A few moments later I delivered the placenta. It was one hour and ten minutes after birth.

It was very exciting the next morning when our $2^{1/2}$ and 4 year-old children came home to meet their baby sister. They held her and kissed her. We've never had any jealousy problem.

I wish every couple could experience the joy and simplicity of a natural homebirth. It's so nice for the baby and it gave our relationship a new depth.

Moonshadow and Aragyn Lutz
Topeka, KS.

THE BIRTH OF GABRIEL ARNTSEN
August 22, 1979
"This Is the Way I Always Wanted It"

My third child was born at home. My first baby, a girl, was born in the hospital. My second baby, also a girl, was born at home with several friends present. This time my husband, Chris, and I were alone.

My family was against my having this homebirth very much, almost as much as they had been against our first one. They just can't understand why we would do such a thing. But we went ahead anyway with our plans. Homebirth seemed so right to us. Besides, they were in Connecticut, and we were in Kansas.

My water started to leak in the morning. I really wasn't sure what it was until evening, when I had to wear Pampers. We realized then what it was and decided to try to get some sleep before labor really started.

<u>Chris:</u> Half of me said, "The baby is coming!" and half of me said, "No!"

There was no way I could sleep, however. Plus, I was so excited. I knew there was going to be nobody else here. There was just Chris and me, and for some reason I got more excited than scared. So, I got up and got things ready and took a shower. By then Chris was up, too, and together we arranged our birthing area in the living room. Funny, unforgettable things happened at this time. For instance, we had no olive oil (for the perineal massage), so Chris decided to liquify some Crisco. But while it was melting we forgot about it, and fifteen minutes later the whole kitchen was smoky!

<u>Chris:</u> I burnt the Hell out of the pan, and had to stick it outdoors, and do a new batch!

The interesting thing was he kept coming back to me and we kept talking. It was just like we didn't have any children. It was just he and I. We turned on the radio and listened to music and relaxed together. It was nice and quiet. We had just one soft light on.

We sterilized the scissors and the shoestrings and got out our sterilized rags, plus a pile of clean diapers. It was about 3:30 or 4 AM, and we were so peaceful. I wasn't even tired.

I had to go to the bathroom several times. I was dripping all the time. But we had a path of newspapers on the floor, so it didn't matter. But every once in a while I'd stop and complain about this leaking, and Chris would say, "Look, don't worry about it! Everything is fine." He always had something positive to say, like, "I can hardly wait! Who cares about the water dripping."

It was so nice, too, that it was just Chris. I wasn't bumping into somebody else.

<u>Chris:</u> This is the way I always wanted it. I could really be myself. No matter how close a friend is, with one there it could never be the same. Birth is an intimate thing.

Previously, when we were thinking about giving birth by ourselves, his sister had said, "But you needed us so badly last time." So, at that time I got to thinking maybe she is right. Maybe I really do need someone there. But then I thought, "Maybe I needed them so badly because they <u>were</u> there! Maybe they were there, and that is why I depended upon them."

Anyway, getting back to the birth, things started to really happen. The water broke. It was just like a balloon. Chris got soaked, but not as badly as with Kiersten's birth. I was surprised that I didn't get sick this time. With my other two babies I threw up.

The contractions were getting closer so Chris went and got the oil about this time and started to do the perineal massage.

<u>Chris:</u> The Crisco was still warm, but it was starting to get solid! It was pretty white by now. [see note, below] Cris was sitting on a pillow on the floor with a couple sofa cushions to her back. As she was slightly elevated it was easier for me to do the perineal massage this time, than last.

During the massage a couple times I got overeager, and started pushing, and Chris slowed me down by telling me if I really didn't need to push, not to. The baby's head was born nice and slowly.

<u>Chris:</u> When the baby's head was completely out I could see the cord on the baby's neck. (It was really just over one shoulder.) So I said, "Easy now, honey, I can see the cord." She was really very much under my control on this coaching thing. So, the baby turned and I told her, "Easy." The cord was hooked over the shoulder, so as the shoulder came out I slid the cord down. It was a little scary.

But Chris didn't get excited or anything. He was very quiet as he suctioned the baby. The baby's body was born with the next contraction, and he started to cry even before his body was completely out. Chris held him briefly, saying, "Honey, it's a boy!"

He didn't nurse right away. Six or seven minutes later the placenta came out. But we didn't out the cord right away. We were in no hurry about anything. I wanted this feeling of euphoria to last.

After Gabe was born it was like - daylight is coming, and the kids are going to get up, and we have to call people. It was just kind of like for those few hours it was just Chris and I, and it was just heaven. Nobody else was around. Nobody else was awake, except the people on the radio. It was a timeless period, and I remember it so well, too.

Chris cleaned up quickly, but about other things we took ever so long. We never even called our parents until about 10 or 11 at night. And I never told my next door neighbor until about six o'clock in the evening. We just wanted to keep this private. We were in no hurry to end it.

Now, wherever I go (at parties, shopping, etc.), I always bring up the subject of homebirth. I can't help it. I will never really know why we had lots of people at Kiersten's birth, because Chris and I had so much love and sharing at Gabriel's birth, it was simply beautiful.

Cris and Chris Arntsen
Edgerton, KS.

[Note: When the Arntsens were telling me about their birth experience and they got to the part about the Crisco turning solid again, I suggested that they leave out the name of the product that they used for the perineal massage. However, they laughingly said, "No. Leave it in!" So, in it is. But, reader, beware! I know nothing about the product and its suitability for increasing the elasticity of the perineum. Olive oil is what is generally used, and it works very nicely.]

SHANNON'S BIRTH
June 12, 1979

After losing my water and being in mild labor for four days, my doctor advised me to go to the hospital for the birth. Larry and I discussed this quite a while. It seems both the baby and I had gone into the high-risk category, because the water had broken, and the doctor really didn't feel safe having us at home. Also, I was delivering about six weeks prematurely.

At 7:00 PM my contractions were becoming quite strong. Larry had told me, with tears in his eyes a few minutes before, that we could go ahead and go to the hospital. I could see he wanted what was best for me and the baby, but he was more disappointed than I had ever seen him.

"I wanted to help you. I wanted to be with you. I wanted to be the one to hold our baby first," he said. I felt like I was cheating him out of his rightful place and that I was hurting him. That's when I decided to stay home. All of a sudden I knew everything was going to be fine for me and our baby.

For the next 10 hours I walked...all over the house, to the front porch and back through the house. I never told Larry where I was going or that I was going most times. I'd just take off. But for each contraction, all I had to do was turn to my right and he was there for me to put my arms around. Generally, we didn't speak. We just held each other.

When we did speak it was whispers in the ear and intimate love talk. Larry didn't miss a contraction. He was there to support me through each one.

When it was time to go into the birth room, Larry continued his support. Had he not been with me I'm sure I would have demanded drugs at that point. But he let me know how loved I was and how close I was getting through it all. He massaged my perineum, smiled at me lovingly, helped me breathe properly, told me he loved me, fluffed my pillows, and made me feel totally safe. There wasn't anything I needed or wanted that wasn't given to me. I was treated like a Princess.

When our son slipped out into Larry's hands and I saw Larry gasp and the tears in his eyes, all of a sudden the room filled with more joy than I had ever experienced. To have been able to see him so overwhelmingly happy gave me more pleasure than even looking at the baby.

Shannon weighed in at 5 pounds, $7^{1/2}$ ounces and was 17 inches long. He is three months old now and has been the happiest, most alert, and most secure of all our babies. (He's our 5th.)

My love for Larry doubled that night. It's possible that Shannon will be our last child. That thought always saddened me before. It doesn't now, because I know that as parents we have given him the best since the beginning...and with the love Larry and I found that night, I know he'll have the best all the way through.

Debbie Miller
Kansas City, MO

The Birth of "The Shan"

We had prepared the birthing room several times in the last week and it would turn out to be false labor. So when Debbie's water broke it was a little unreal to me that birth was imminent.

It didn't happen that night, however. We went to the

doctor's the following day (Saturday) and she said it would be sometime that night. It wasn't, or the next day, either.

We were pretty disappointed and went to see the doctor on Monday. We were advised to go to the hospital because it had been so long since the water had broken and the baby was a few weeks premature. We went home and laid around pretty much feeling the effect of our disappointment.

A friend of ours called me and told me to basically carry through on what we wanted without counter-intention on it. After that Debbie and I really talked to each other about our considerations on this birth and really let each other know how we felt.

Shortly afterward Shannon decided to be born and hard labor began. There was twelve hours of it. We walked and danced. We even had time for a little love making in the candlelight.

Through the night I checked several times to see how much Debbie had dilated. I've never been prouder of a Lady than that night and morning. As the time grew closer, I used the perineal massage described in the homebirth data that we had been given. Talking was kept to a minimum.

Through all of this our friend, Diane, was there helping whenever asked, but never interfering in the intimacy of it.

When the baby's head crowned and I thought, "What do I do?" Diane let me know in a whisper.

I applied no pressure to the baby's head, and there was no jerking or pulling at all. The next thing I knew, Shannon was in my arms and in three seconds he cried out as if to let me know he was OK. I held him for a moment, then put him on his mother's stomach.

The moment was like I had never experienced. I was overwhelmed with joy and felt like "We Did It!"...and thankful to my Lady and filled with admiration and respect for her. The rest of the morning was like an 'after glow.'

My deepest thanks go to our friends who spoke the truth and understood, to my Lady for the gift of this experience, and to Shannon for picking us.

Larry Miller

THE END

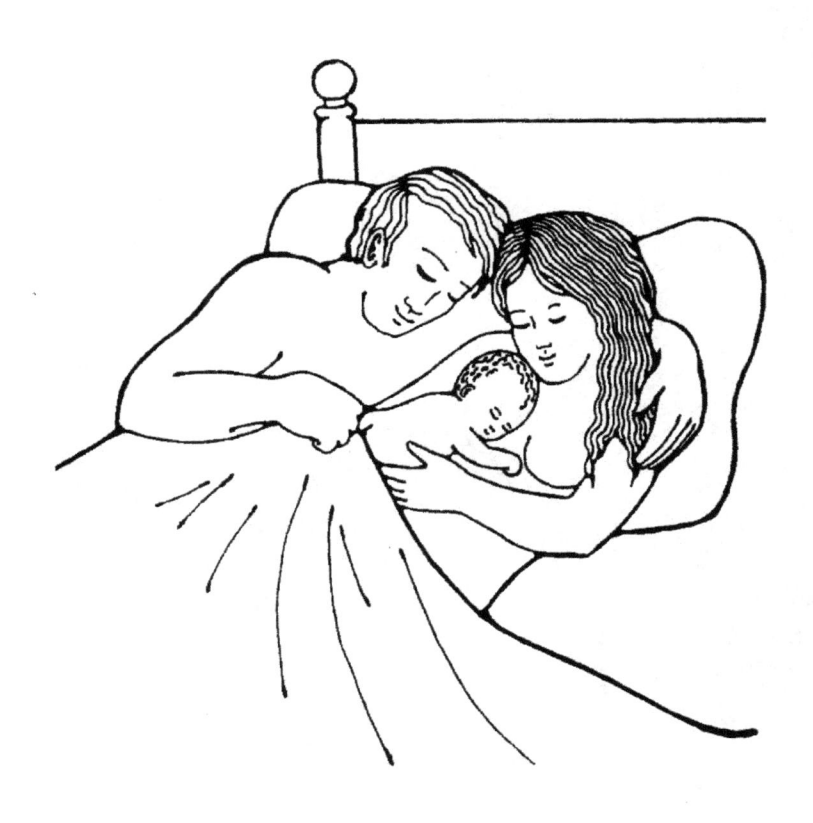

NOTES

Chapter 1

1. Grantly Dick-Read. 1970. *Childbirth Without Fear.* New York, Harper & Row, Perennial Library Edition, p. 34.
2. Sheila Kitzinger. 1967. *The Experience of Childbirth.* Baltimore, Penguin-Pelican, p. 248.
3. N. Kalichman, M.D. 1951. "On Some Psychological Aspects of the Management of Labor," *Psychiatric Quarterly*, Vol 25: No. 4, p. 655-671.
4. Niles Newton, PhD. 1955. *Maternal Emotions.* New York, Paul B. Hoeber, Co., p. 87.
5. Masters and Johnson. 1966. *Human Sexual Response.* Boston, Little, Brown & Co., p. 275.
6. Jessica Dick-Read. 1965. London, William Heinemann Medical Books, Ltd., [This flush is called the Malar flush]
7. William H. Masters &Virginia E. Johnson. op.cit., p.33, 299.
8. Sheila Kitzinger. op.cit., p. 157.
9. Sheila Kitzinger. 1977. *Education and Counseling for Childbirth.* London, Baillere Tindall, p. 185.
10. Masters and Johnson. op.cit., p. 118.
11. Moonshadow and Aragyn Lutz. 1978. "The Best Way to Have a Baby," *The New Nativity.* Vol. 11, No. 4, Winter, p. 2. It is reprinted in this book starting on p. 189.

12. Masters and Johnson. op.cit., p. 5.

13. Leon Chertok. 1973. *Motherhood and Personality*. New York, Harper & Row, Barnes & Noble Import Division, p. 29.

14. Robert A. Bradley, M.D. 1965. *Husband-Coached Childbirth*. New York, Harper & Row, p. 67.

15. Margaret Mead. 1967. "Cultural Patterning," *Childbearing: Its Social and Psychological Aspects*. Richardson and Guttmacher, eds. Baltimore, Williams & Wilkins Co., p. 173.

16. Dr. Walter Menninger. July 12, 1976. "Home Childbirth Has Its Value," *Kansas City Star*.

17. Andre Hellegers, M.D. Sept. 13, 1975. "Compassion With Competence," *America*, p. 114.

18. Waldo Fielding, M.D. 1971. *Pregnancy: The Best State of the Union*. New York, Crowell Co., p. 134.

19. Robert E. Hall, M.D. Feb. 27, 1967. *New York Times*.

20. William J. Sweeney, III, M.D. with Barbara Lang Stern. 1973. *Woman's Doctor*. New York, William Morrow & Co., p. 33.

21. Gerald Jonas. March, 1969. "Diary of an Expectant Father," *Family Circle*, p. 90.

Chapter 2

1. Pat Kilcoyne. May-June, 1967. "From a Happy Father in Chicago," *LaLeche League News*, p. 6.

2. Bob Yoho. March 2, 1974. "Home Birth," *Hutchinson (KS.) News*.

3. Tonya Brooks. August, 1974. "Childbirth - the Psychological Issues," *The East West Journal*. Vol. 4:7, p. 24.

4. Niles Newton, Ph.D. 1955. *Maternal Emotions*. New York, Paul B, Hoeber Co., p. 87. Also see - Newton, N. Sept. 1968. "The Effects of Disturbance on Labor," *American Journal of Obstetrics and Gynecology*, 101: 1096-1102.

5. Neil Collins. 1976. "Birth in a Grocery Store," *Safe Alternatives in Childbirth*. Stewart & Stewart, eds., Chapel Hill, N.C., NAPSAC, p. 153.

6. Cedar Koons. "Homebirth: A Family Awakening," ibid., p. 145.

Chapter 3

1. *Emergency Childbirth*. 1966. U.S. Government Printing Office, 0-220-818.
2. Gregory L. Hack. Jan. 9, 1976. "Baby Comes into Cold World," *Kansas City Times*, p. 10A.
3. *Emergency Childbirth*, op.cit.
4. John D.W. Hunter, M.D. Fall, 1974. "A Look at High Risk Pregnancy," *Birth and the Family Journal*, p. 15.
5. Lester Hazell. 1974. *Birth Goes Home*. Seattle, Catalyst Publishing Co.
6. Constance A. Bean. 1972. *Methods of Childbirth*. New York, Doubleday, p. 124.
7. John Bowlby, M.D. 1969. "Attachment and Loss," *Attachment*, Vol. 1. New York, Basic Books.
8. Janet Adler. "The Study of an Autistic Child," from the proceedings of one of the early ADTA conferences, pgs. 43-48. Available from, American Dance Therapy Association, Suite 210, 1000 Century Plaza, Columbia, MD. 21044.
9. Barry Neil Kaufman. 1976. *Son-Rise*. New York, Harper & Row, p. 39.
10. J. P. Scott. Feb. 9, 1968. "Phenotype: Postnatal Development," *Science*, p. 658.
11. John Bowlby, M.D. op.cit., p. 168.
12. Aljean Harmetz. Feb. 1972. "The Way Childbirth Really Is," *Today's Health*, p. 31.
13. Robert A. Bradley, M.D. 1965. *Husband-Coached Childbirth*, New York, Harper & Row, p. 18.
14. Marshall H. Klaus, M.D., et al. March 2, 1972. "Maternal Attachment," *New England Journal of Medicine*, p. 460-463.
15. John H. Kennell, M.D., et al. April, 1974. "Maternal Behavior One Year After Early and Extended Post-partum Contact," *Developmental Medicine and Child Neurology*, pp.

172-179.

16. Marshall Klaus, M.D. op.cit., p. 462.

17. Marshall H. Klaus, M.D., et al. Aug. 1970. "Human Maternal Behavior at the First Contact With Her Young," *Pediatrics*, p. 188.

18. Kenneth S. Robson. Vol. 8, 1967. "The Role of Eye-to-eye Contact in Maternal-Infant Attachment," *Journal of Child Psychology and Psychiatry*, pp. 13-25.

19. Eckhard H. Hess. April, 1965. "Attitude and Pupil Size," *Scientific American*, pp. 46-54.

20. Marietta Dunn. Dec. 3, 1975. "Newborn's First Hours Building Blocks of Family," *Kansas City Times*, p. 16A.

Chapter 4

1. Thaddeus L. Montgomery, M.D. 1958, Vol. 76. "Physiologic Considerations in Labor and the Puerperium," *American Journal of Obstetrics and Gynecology*, pp. 706-715.

2. William J. Sweeney, III, M.D. April, 1973. "Woman's Doctor," *Readers Digest*, p. 254. Condensed from Woman's Doctor, by William J. Sweeney, III, M.D., with Barbara Lang Stern. New York, William Morrow & Co., p. 53.

3. Doris Haire. 1972. *Cultural Warping of Childbirth*, International Childbirth Education Association, p. 11.

4. Constance A. Bean. 1972. *Methods of Childbirth*, Garden City, N.Y., Doubleday, p. 128.

5. Watson A. Bowes, Jr., M.D. June, 1970. "Obstetrical Medication and Infant Outcome: A Review of the Literature," *The Effects of Obstetrical Medication on Fetus and Infant, Monographs of the Society for Research in Child Development*, Serial 137, Vol. 35:4, p. 16.

6. Watson A. Bowes, Jr., M.D., ibid.

7. Elliott H. McCleary. 1974. *New Miracles of Childbirth*. New York, David McKay Co., p. 100.

8. William F. Windle. Oct., 1969. "Brain Damage by Asphyxia at Birth," *Scientific American*, pp. 77-84.

9. Marge Holler Stephens. Dec. 2, 1975. "Complications

Concern Doctors," *Kansas City Star*, p. 10.

10. T. Berry Brazelton, M.D. June, 1970. "What Makes a Good Father," *Redbook*, p. 121.

11. "Birth of an Abnormal Baby," Oct., 1975. *Kansas ICEA Newsletter*, p. 4.

Chapter 5

1. Waldo L. Fielding, M.D. 1971. *Pregnancy: The Best State of the Union*. New York, Crowell Co., p. 143.

2. Bete Gillespie. Dec., 1969. " 'Fathers Only' Journals," *Today's Health*, p. 16-17.

3. Frederick Leboyer, M.D. 1975. *Birth Without Violence* New York, Alfred A. Knopf.

4. Jacques Lowe. 1961. *Portrait - The Emergence of John F. Kennedy*. New York, McGraw-Hill, p. 51.

5. Katherine Burton. 1937. *Sorrow Built a Bridge*. New York, Longmans, Green & Co., p. 112.

6. Arthur D. and Libby L. Colman. 1971. *Pregnancy: The Psychological Experience*. New York, Herder & Herder, p. 112.

7. Neil Collins, J.D. 1976. "Birth in a Grocery Store," *Safe Alternatives in Childbirth*. Stewart & Stewart, eds. Chapel Hill, NC, NAPSAC, pp. 149,150.

8. Robert A. Bradley, M.D. Nov. - Dec., 1962. "Fathers Presence in Delivery Rooms," *Psychosomatics*. Vol. III, No. 6.

9. Robert Brizzolara. Dec., 1968. "Maverick Physician," *St. Anthony Messenger*, p. 13.

10. Gerald Jonas. March, 1969. "Diary of an Expectant Father," *Family Circle*, p. 90.

11. Charlotte Ward and Fred Ward. 1976. *The Home Birth Book*. Wash., D.C., Inscape Publishers, p.115.

12. Rita Kramer. July 11, 1976. "Revolution in the Delivery Room," *New York Times Magazine*, p. 18.

13. Patricia Corrigan Krauska. Jan. 15, 1976. "Some Mothers Prefer Home Births," *St. Louis Globe Democrat*, p. 1B

14. Dorothy V. Whipple, M.D. Oct., 1965.

"Breastfeeding in Today's World," *Journal of the American Medical Women's Association,* pp. 936-937.

15. J. Bronowski. 1973. *The Ascent of Man,* Boston, Little, Brown & Co., p. 116.

Chapter 6

1. "Spiritual Midwifery." 1974. *Hey Beatnik!* Summertown, TN, The Book Publishing Co.
2. Ina May Gaskin. 1978. *Spiritual Midwifery.* Summertown, TN, The Book Publishing Co., p. 52.
3. "Mister Midwife." June, 1972. *Prevention.*
4. "Special Delivery." July 30, 1973. *Newsweek,* p. 75.
5. Margaret Gamper, R.N. 1971. *Preparation for the Heir Minded.* Chicago, Midwest Parentcraft Center, p. 46.
6. Sheila Kitzinger. 1967. *Experience of Childbirth.* Baltimore, Penguin-Pelican, p. 136.
7. Margaret Mead & Niles Newton. 1967. "Cultural Patterning of Perinatal Behavior." *Childbearing: Its Psychological and Social Aspects,* Guttmacher & Richardson, eds. Baltimore, Williams & Wilkins Co.
8. Ina May Gaskin. Jan. 1977. *Proceedings of the Midwives Conference,* El Paso, Texas.
9. A. Jhirad, M.D., and T. Vago, M.D. March, 1973. "Induction of Labor by Breast Stimulation." *Obstetrics & Gynecology,* p. 350.
10. "Emergency Childbirth." Fall, 1976. *News from H.O.M.E.,* p. 5.
11. William H. Hazlett, M.D. "The Husband at Delivery." *Marriage,* pp. 46-47.
12. Robert Bahr. Feb., 1975. "A New Joy for Parents: Let Dad Deliver the Baby." *Prevention,* p. 73.
13. Carolyn Butwin. May-June 1972. "Daddy-delivered." *LaLeche League News,* p. 34.
14. Marge Holler Stevens,. Dec. 1, 1975. "Childbirth in Homes." *Kansas City Star,* p. 12.
15. Robert A. Bradley, M.D. 1965. *Husband-Coached Childbirth,* New York, Harper & Row, p. 79.

16. "A Statement on Abortion by One-hundred Professors of Obstetrics." April 1, 1972. *American Journal of Obstetrics and Gynecology*, p. 992.

APPENDIX

SUGGESTED READING LIST

The following books will be helpful for anyone planning to give birth at home:

Emergency Childbirth, Gregory White, M. D.
Childbirth at Home, Marion Sousa
The Joy of Natural Childbirth, Helen Wessel.
Home Oriented Maternity Experience, the H.O.M.E. manual
Spiritual Midwifery, Ina May Gaskin
Birth Book, Raven Lang
The Womanly Art of Breastfeeding, LaLeche League
HAPPY BIRTH DAYS, Marilyn A. Moran, ed.

The following books don't mention birth, specifically, but they can help you have a better experience:

Touching, the Human Significance of the Skin, A. Montagu
Total Massage, Jack Hofer

Also of interest:

Experience of Childbirth, Sheila Kitzinger
Commonsense Childbirth, Lester Hazell
Husband-Coached Childbirth, Robert Bradley, M. D.
Cultural Warping of Childbirth, Doris Haire
Nourishing Your Unborn Child, Phyllis Williams
Diet for a Small Planet, F.M. Lappe

BIBLIOGRAPHY

Bibliography - Books

Anderson, H.H., ed. *Creativity and its Cultivation.* 1959. NY, Harper.

Arasteh, A. Reza. 1965. *Final Integration in the Adult Personality.* Leiden, Netherlands, E.J. Brill.

Ardrey, Robert. 1970. *Social Contract.* N.Y., Atheneum.

Ardrey, Robert. 1966. *The Territorial Imperative.* N.Y., Dell.

Arms, Suzanne. *Immaculate Deception.* 1975. Boston, Houghton Mifflin Co.

Asimov, Isaac. *Life and Energy.* 1962. Garden City, NY, Doubleday & Co.

Bean, Constance A. 1972. *Methods of Childbirth.* Garden City, NY, Doubleday & Co.

Birdwhistell, R. L. 1970. *Kinesics and Context.* Philadelphia, Univ. of Penn. Press.

Bowes, W., et al. June 1970. "The Effects of Obstetrical Medication on Fetus and Infant," *Monographs of the Society for Research on Child Development.* Vol. 35, No 187.

Bowlby, John, M.D. 1969. *Attachment and Loss.* N.Y., Basic Books. Vol. I, II & III.

Bradley, Robert A. , M.D. 1965. *Husband-Coached Childbirth.* N.Y. Harper & Row.

Brewer, Thomas A., M.D. 1966. *Metabolic Toxemia of Late*

Pregnancy. Springfield, IL. Charles C. Thomas.

Bronowski, J. 1973. *The Ascent of Man.* Boston, Little Brown.

Burton, Katherine. 1937. *Sorrow Built a Bridge.* NY, Longman's Green & Co.

Carpenter, Edmund, and Marshall McLuhan, eds. 1968. *Explorations in Communication.* Boston, Beacon Press.

Carter, Patricia C. 1957. *Come Gently, Sweet Lucina.* Titusville, FL, Patricia Cloyd Carter.

Chabon, Irwin, M.D. 1966. *Awake and Aware.* NY, Delacorte.

Chertok, Leon. 1973. *Motherhood and Personality.* NY, Harper & Row.

Christman, R. J. 1971. *Sensory Experience.*

Cohen, Allen. 1971. *Childbirth is Ecstasy.* San Francisco, Aquarius.

Colman, Arthur D. and Libby L. Colman. 1971. *Pregnancy: the Psychological Experience.* NY, Herder & Herder.

Daniel-Rops, Henri, Michel Riquet, Gustave Thibon, Jacques Madaule. 1964. *Love is Forever.* Dublin, Scepter.

Dantec, Francois. 1963. *Love is Life.* Notre Dame, IN, Univ. of Notre Dame Press.

Davis, Adelle. 1973. *Let's Have Healthy Children.* NY, Harcourt Brace Jovanovich.

de Lubac, Henri, Teilhard deChardin. 1965. *The Man and His Meaning.* NY, The New American Library.

Deutsch, Helene. 1945. "Motherhood," *Psychology of Women.* NY, Grune & Stratton, Vol. 2.

Deutsch, Roland M. 1968. *The Key to Feminine Response in Marriage.* NY, Ballantine Books.

Devaux, Andre. 1968. *Teilhard and Womanhood.* NY, Paulist Press.

Dick-Read, Grantly.1944. *Childbirth Without Fear.* NY, Harper.

Dick-Read, Jessica. 1965. *What Every Woman Should Know about Childbirth.* London, William Heineman Medical Books.

Dobzhansky, Theodosius. 1956. *Biological Basis of Human Freedom.* NY, Columbia Univ. Press.

Dobzhansky, Theodosius. 1964. *Heredity and the Nature of Man.* NY, Harcourt, Brace.

Dubarle, Andre-Marie. 1964. *The Biblical Doctrine of Original Sin.* NY. Herder & Herder.

Dubos, Rene. 1972. *A God Within.* NY, Scribners.

Dubos, Rene. 1965. *Man Adapting* New Haven, Yale Univ. Press.

Eloesser, Leo, et al. 1959. *Pregnancy, Childbirth and the Newborn: A Manual for Rural Midwives.* Mexico City, Instituto Indigenista Interamericano.

Emergency Childbirth. U.S. Govt. Printing Office, 1966-0-220-818

Erikson. Erik H. 1963. *Childhood and Society.* NY, Norton.

Fast. J. 1970. *Body Language.* NY, M. Evans.

Fielding, Waldo. 1971. *Pregnancy: the Best State of the Union.* NY, Crowell Co.

Flanagan, Geraldine Lux. 1962. *The First Nine Months of Life.* NY, Simon & Schuster.

Francoer, Robert T. 1965. *Perspectives in Evolution.* Baltimore, MD, Helicon.

Francoer, Robert T. 1961. *The World of Teilhard.* Baltimore, MD, Helicon.

Gamper, Margaret, R.N. 1971. *Preparation for the Heir Minded.* Chicago, Midwest Parentcraft Center.

Gaskin, Ina May. 1978. *Spiritual Midwifery.* Summertown, TN, Book Publishing Co.

Gaskin, Stephen. 1974. *Hey Beatnik!* Summertown, TN, Book Pub. Co.

Guitton, Jean. 1965. *Feminine Fulfillment.* Chicago, IL, Franciscan Herald Press.

Guitton, Jean. 1966. *Human Love.* Chicago, IL, Franciscan Herald Press.

Guttmacher, Alan F., M.D. 1973. *Pregnancy, Birth and Family Planning* NY, Viking Press.

Haire, Doris. 1972. *The Cultural Warping of Childbirth.* Minneapolis, International Childbirth Education Association.

Hall, E.T. 1959. *The Silent Language.* Garden City, Doubleday.

Hazell, Lester. 1974. *Birth Goes Home.* Seattle, Catalyst Pub.

Hazell, Lester. 1969. *Commonsense Childbirth.* NY, G.P. Putnams's Sons.

Hofer, Jack. 1976. *Total Massage.* NY, Grosset & Dunlap.

Holmes, Marjorie. 1974. *Two From Galilee.* NY, Bamtam.

Howell, Mary C., M.D. 1975. *Helping Ourselves: Families and the Human Network.* Boston, MA, Beacon.

Jourard, Sidney M. 1964. *The Transparent Self.* Princeton, NJ, D. Van Nostrand.

Kaufman, Barry Neil. 1976. *Son-Rise.* NY, Harper & Row.

Kitzinger, Sheila. 1977. *Education and Counseling for Childbirth.* London, Baillere Tindall.

Kitzinger, Sheila. 1972. *Experience of Childbirth.* Baltimore, MD, Penguin.

Klaus, Marshall H., M.D. and John H. Kennell, M.D. 1976.

Maternal-infant Bonding. St. Louis, MO, Vosby.

Lang, Raven. 1972. *Birth Book.* Ben Lomond, CA, Genesis.

Leboyer, Frederick, M.D. 1975. *Birth Without Violence.* NY, Knopf.

Leboyer, Frederick, M.D. 1976. *Loving Hands.* NY, Knopf.

Lepp, Ignace. 1963. *The Psychology of Loving* NY, New American Library.

Lowe, Jacques. 1961. *Portrait: The Emergence of John F. Kennedy.* NY, McGraw-Hill.

Masters, William H. and Virginia E. Johnson. 1966. *Human Sexual Response.* Boston, MA, Little Brown & Co.

May, Rollo. 1953. *Man's Search for Himself.* NY, Norton.

McCleary, Elliott H. 1974. *New Miracles of Childbirth.* NY, David McKay Co.

McDonagh, Enda. 1963. *The Meaning of Christian Marriage.* NY, Alba House.

Mead, Margaret. 1949. *Male and Female*. NY, Morrow.

Meltzer, David. 1967. *Journal of the Birth*. Berkeley, Oyez Press.

Milinaire, Caterine. 1974. *Birth*. NY, Harmony Books.

Montagu, Ashley. 1961. *Life Before Birth*. NY, New American Library.

Montagu, Ashley. 1978. *Touching: The Human Significance of the Skin*. NY, Harper.

Newton, Eric. 1962. *The Meaning of Beauty*. Baltimore, MD, Penguin.

Newton, Niles. 1955. *Maternal Emotions*. NY, Paul B. Hoeber.

Nogar, Raymond P. 1963. *Wisdom of Evolution*. Garden City, NY, Doubleday.

Oraison, Marc. 1958. *Man and Wife*. NY, Macmillan.

Oraison, Marc. 1967. *The Human Mystery of Sexuality*. NY, Sheed & Ward.

Overstreet, Bonaro W. 1951. *Understanding Fear in Ourselves and Others*. NY, Harper & Row.

Pfeiffer, John. 1955. *The Human Brain*. NY, Harper.

Powell, John, S.J. 1967. *Why Am I Afraid to Love?* Chicago, IL, Argus.

Rock, Augustine. 1966. *Sex, Love, and the Life of the Spirit*. Chicago, IL, Priory Press.

Russell, E.S. 1945. *The Directiveness of Organic Activities*. London, Cambridge Univ. Press.

Schillebeeckx, Edward. 1963. *Christ: The Sacrament of the Encounter with God*. NY, Sheed & Ward.

Schoonenberg, Piet. 1965. *Man and Sin*. Univ. of Notre Dame Pr.

Selye, Hans. 1956. *The Stress of Life*. NY, McGraw-Hill.

Sousa, Marion. 1976. *Childbirth at Home*. Englewood Cliffs, NJ, Prentice Hall.

Stern, Karl, M.D. 1965. *Flight from Woman*. NY, Farrar, Straus.

Stewart, David and Lee Stewart, eds. 1979. *Compulsory Hospitalization*. Marble Hill, MO, NAPSAC, Vol. I, II & III.

Stewart, David and Lee Stewart, eds. 1976. *Safe*

Alternatives in Childbirth. NAPSAC.

Stewart, David and Lee Stewart, eds. 1977. *21st Century Obstetrics, Now!* NAPSAC, Vol. I & II.

Sweeney, William J., III, M.D., with Barbara Lang Stern. 1973. *Woman's Doctor.* NY, William Morrow & Co.

Tanzer, Deborah, and Jean L. Block. 1972. *Why Natural Childbirth.* Garden City, NY, Doubleday & Co.

Teilhard de Chardin, Pierre. 1960. *The Divine Milieu.* NY, Harper.

Teilhard de Chardin, Pierre. 1962. *Human Energy.* NY, Harcourt Brace Jovanovich.

The Womanly Art of Breastfeeding. 1963. Franklin Park, IL, LaLeche League, International.

Thibon, Gustave. 1952. *What God Has Joined Together.* Chicago, IL, Henry Regnery Co.

Vellay, Pierre, M.D. 1969. *Childbirth with Confidence.* NY, Macmillan.

Ward, Barbara and Rene Dubos. 1972. *Only One Earth.* NY, W.W. Norton & Co.

Ward, Charlotte and Fred Ward. 1976. *The Home Birth Book.* Washington, D.C., Inscape Pub.

Wertz, Richard W. and Dorothy C. 1977. *Lying-In: A History of Childbirth in America.* NY, The Free Press.

Wessel, Helen. 1963. *Natural Childbirth and the Christian Family.* NY, Harper & Row.

White, Gregory J., M.D. 1968. *Emergency Childbirth.* Franklin, Park, IL, Police Training Foundation.

Masterpieces of Painting in the Metropolitan Museum of Art. Comments by E. Standen & T. Folds. NY Graphic Society, p.25

Bibliography — Articles

Adler, Janet. "The Study of an Autistic Child," from proceedings of one of the early ADTA (American Dance Therapy Association) conferences.

Allen, Carroll. May, 1975. "Let's Put the Joy and Dignity Back into Birthing," *Homemakers Magazine.* Toronto, pp. 18-

22.
Allen, Carroll. Spring, 1975. "An Obstetrician Teaches Dad to Deliver his Baby Himself," *People,* pp. 40-43.

Anonymous. May, 1954. "Born in the Bathtub," *Child & Family Digest,* p. 86.

"A Statement on Abortion by One-hundred Professors of Obstetrics," *American Journal of Obstetrics & Gynecology.* April 1, 1972, p. 992

"At-home Delivery - A New Trend to an Old Idea," *Life.* Aug. 18, 1972.

Bahr, Robert. Feb., 1975. "A New Joy for Parents: Let Dad Deliver the Baby," *Prevention,* p. 73.

Bing, Elizabeth and Libby Colman. Nov., 1977. "Sex During Pregnancy," *Redbook,* p. 89.

Birdwhistell, Ray L. 1960. "Kinesics and Communication," *Explorations in Communication.* Carpenter and McLuhan, eds. Boston, MA, Beacon.

"Birth of an Abnormal Baby," *Kansas ICEA Newsletter.* Oct. 1975.

"Boys Deliver Mother's Baby." Nov. 12, 1977. Newspaper article, source unknown.

Brackbill, Y. et al. Feb. 1, 1974. "Obstetric Premedication and Infant Outcome," *American Journal of Obstetrics and Gynecology,* pp. 377-384

Bradley, Robert A., M.D. Nov.-Dec., 1962. "Fathers Presence in Delivery Rooms," *Psychosomatics.*

Brazelton, T. Berry, M.D. April 1961. "Psychophysiologic Reactions in the Neonate: The Effect of Maternal Medication on the Neonate and His Behavior," *Journal of Pediatrics,* pp.513-518.

Brazelton, T. Berry, M.D. June 1970. "What Makes a Good Father," *Redbook.*

Brazelton, T. Berry, M.D. February, 1971. "What Childbirth Drugs Can do to Your Child," *Redbook.*

Breeden, Nancy. Jan.-Feb. 1978. "Sex and Breastfeeding," *La Leche League News,* p. 4.

Bridge, Peter. Nov. 9, 1974. "1,000 Midwife Dads do it Themselves," *National Star,* p. 12.

Brizzolara, Robert. Dec. 1968. "Maverick Physician," *St. Anthony Messenger*, pp. 11-16.

Brooks, Tonya. Aug. 1974. "Childbirth: The Psychological Issues," *The East West Journal*, p. 24.

Buchwald, Art. Feb. 6, 1980. "Turn-about," *Overland Park (KS) Sun*, p. 4.

Butwin, Carolyn. May-June 1972. "Daddy-delivered," *La Leche League News*, p. 34.

Collins, Neil. 1976. "Birth in a Grocery Store," *Safe Alternatives in Childbirth*. Stewart & Stewart, eds, NAPSAC.

de Mille, Agnes. 1962. "The Milk of Paradise," *American Women: The Changing Image,* ed. B. Cassara. Boston, MA, Beacon.

Dunn, Marietta. Dec. 3, 1975. "Newborn's First Hours Building Blocks of Family," *Kansas City Times*, p. 15A.

Egginton, Joyce. June 10, 1973. "Have Your Babies the Native Way," *The Observer (London)*.

"Emergency Childbirth," *News from H.O.M.E.*, Fall,1976, p. 5.

"Extractor Called Safer as Birth Aid," *Stamford (CT) Advocate,* Dec. 29, 1972.

Fisher, Kathlin. April 9, 1972. "Home Delivery," *The Plain Dealer.* Cleveland, OH.

"Four Mental Patients Assist in a Birth: Mother and Baby Did Fine!" *New York Times*, Nov. 17, 1976, p. A24.

Fraley, Pierre C. Sept.-Oct., 1959. "Hour's Delay in Cutting the Cord Gives Babies a Healthier Start," *Child-Family Digest*, pp. 54-56.

Frank, Lawrence K. "Tactile Communication," *Explorations in Communication.* Carpenter & McLuhan, eds., op.cit.

Gaskin, Ina May. Jan. 1977. *Proceedings of Midwives Conference*, El Paso, Texas.

Gillespie, Bete. Dec. 1969. " 'Fathers Only' Journals," *Today's Health,* pp. 16-17.

Goodman, Ellen. Aug. 27. 1969. "Why I Had My Baby at Home," *Boston Globe.*

Graham, Jory. 1978. "Home is Where We Want to Be,"

Chicago Daily News.

Greenberg, Martin, M.D. and Norman Morris, M.D. July 1974. "Engrossment: The Newborn's Impact Upon the Father," *American Journal of Orthopsychiatry*, pp. 520-531.

Hack, Gregory L. Jan. 9, 1976. "Baby Comes into Cold World," *Kansas City Times*, p. 10A.

Haggerty, Joan. Dec. 1972 or Jan. 1973. "Childbirth Made Difficult," *Ms.*

Haley, Jean. Dec. 4, 1977. "Born at Home," *Kansas City Star*, p.12.

Hall, Robert E., M.D. Feb. 27, 1967. *NY Times*.

Harmetz, Aljean. Feb. 1972. "The Way Childbirth Really Is," *Today's Health*, p. 29.

Hart, Scarlett. Winter, 1977. "A Lingering Sweetness," *The New Nativity*, p. 5

Hazlett, William H., M.D. "The Husband at Delivery," *Marriage*, pp. 39-47.

Hazlett, William H., M.D. Fall, 1967. "The Male Factor in Obstetrics," *Child & Family*, p. 3.

Hellegers, Andre, M.D. Sept. 13, 1975. "Compassion with Competence," *America*, p. 114.

Hess, Eckhard H. April, 1965. "Attitude and Pupil Size," *Scientific American,* pp. 46-54.

Hess, Eckhard H. May 10, 1971. "Home Delivery," *Newsweek*, p. 104.

Hunter, John D.W., M.D. Fall, 1974. "A Look at High Risk Pregnancy," *Birth and the Family Journal*, p. 15.

Hunter, John D.W., M.D. Aug. 22, 1976. "I Gave Birth at Home," *Awake,* p. 20.

Jhirad, A., M.D, and T. Vago, M.D. March, 1973, "Induction of Labor by Breast Stimulation," *Obstetrics and Gynecology*, p. 350.

Jonas, Gerald. March, 1969. "Diary of an Expectant Father," *Family Circle*, p. 90.

Kalichman, N., M.D. 1951. "On Some Psychological Aspects of the Management of Labor," *Psychiatric Quarter*, Vol. 25:4, p.655.

Kapel, Saul, M.D. April 29, 1975. "Fatherly Bond

Strong at Birth," *Kansas City Star*, p. 22.

Kennell, John H., M.D., et al. April, 1974. "Maternal Behavior One Year After Early and Extended Postpartum Contact," *Developmental Medicine & Child Neurology*, pp. 172-179.

Kilcoyne, Patrick. May-June, 1967. "From a Happy Father in Chicago," *La Leche League News*, p. 6.

Klaus, Marshall H., M.D., and John H. Kennell, M.D. Nov., 1970. "Mothers Separated from their Newborn Infants," *Pediatric Clinics of North America*, pp. 1015-1035.

Klaus, Marshall H., M.D., and John H. Kennell, M.D. Aug., 1970. "Human Maternal Behavior at the First Contact with Her Young," *Pediatrics*, pp. 187-191.

Klaus, Marshall H., M.D., and John H. Kennell, M.D. March 2, 1972. "Maternal Attachment," *New England Journal of Medicine*.

Klemesrud, Judy. Nov. 9, 1971. "Giving Birth at Home: A Great Experience or Step Backward?" *NY Times*, p. 56.

Kramer, Rita. July 11, 1976. "Revolution in the Delivery Room," *NY Times Magazine*, p. 18.

Krauska, Patricia Corrigan. Jan. 15, 1976. "Some Mothers Prefer Home Births," *St. Louis Globe Democrat*, p. 1B.

Leighton, Sally. May-June, 1956. "Childbirth Reconsidered," *Child-Family Digest*, pp. 84-89.

Lopez, Barry. Oct., 1974. "Being Born at Home is Wonderful," *Lady's Circle*, p. 27.

Lutz, Moonshadow. Winter, 1978. "The Best Way to Have a Baby," *The New Nativity*.

Marshall, Margaret Curtin. Sept. 1974. "My Husband Delivered our Baby," *Good Housekeeping*, pp. 77-80.

Maslow, Abraham. 1975. "Love in Healthy People," *The Practice of Love*, A. Montagu, ed., Englewood Cliffs, NJ, Prentice Hall, p.112.

McCann, Jean. June 1971. "They Want to Have Their Babies at Home," *Marriage*, p. 10.

Mead, Margaret and Niles Newton. 1967. "Cultural Patterning of Perinatal Behavior," *Childbearing: Its Social and*

Psychological Aspects, Richardson & Guttmacher, eds., Baltimore, MD, Williams & Wilkins Co.

Menninger, Walter, M.D. July 12, 1976. "Home Childbirth has its Value," *Kansas City Star*, 1976.

Menninger, Walter, M.D. Nov. 22, 1976. "Mothers Bond with Baby Affected by Early Contact," *Kansas City Star*, p. 8.

Montagu, Ashley, M.D. May-June, 1958. "Personal Histories of Natural Childbirth," *Child-Family Digest*, p. 92.

Montagu, Ashley, M.D. March, 1956. "Babies Should be Born at Home!," *Child-Family Digest*, pp. 64-78. Reprinted from *Ladies Home Journal*, Aug. 1955.

Montgomery, Thaddeus L., M.D. 1958. "Physiologic Considerations in Labor and the Puerperium," *American Journal of Obstetrics & Gynecology*, Vol.76 pp. 706-715.

Mordecai, Mary Day. July 28, 1974. "Families Revive Home Birth Custom to Share Experience," *The News and Observer* (Raleigh, NC), p. 2-III.

Newton, N. Sept. 1968. "The Effects of Disturbance of Labor," *American Journal of Obstetrics & Gynecology*, pp. 1096-1102.

Newton, N. April 15, 1971. "New Vertical Delivery is Turning Obstetrics Upside Down," *Daily News* (Springfield, MA).

O'Neill, Michael. Sept.-Oct., 1958. "The Super-germ that Menaces Hospitals," *Child-Family Digest*, pp. 31-37.

Robinson, Michael A. March 2, 1979. "Infant Born in Speeding Car," *Kansas City Times*.

Robson, Kenneth S. 1967. "The Role of Eye-to-eye Contact in Maternal-infant Attachment," *Journal of Child Psychology & Psychiatry*, Vol. 8, pp. 13-25.

Rutstein, David D., M.D. Aug., 1964. "Why Do We Let These Babies Die," [Ten other countries have lower infant-mortality rates than the U.S], *Readers Digest*, pp. 56-57.

Scott, J. P. Feb. 9, 1968. "Phenotype: Postnatal Development," *Science*, p. 658.

"Special Delivery," *Newsweek*, July 30, 1973, p. 75.

Stein, Ruthe. June 29, 1973. "Where Should Babies be

Born?" *San Francisco Chronicle*, p. 24.

Stephens, Marge Holler. Dec. 1, 1975. "Childbirths in Homes: Hospitals not 'Natural,' " *Kansas City Star*, p. 12.

Stephens, Marge Holler. Dec.2, 1975. "Complications Concern Doctors," *Kansas City Star*, p. 10.

"The New Fathers: Fatherhood Begins at the Moment of Birth," *Life*, July 14, 1972, p. 69.

Thompson, Nancy. Nov. 16, 1972. "Homebirth is a Spiritual Experience," *The News Sun* (Cleveland, OH), p. 2B.

Van Dellen, Dr. Theodore. Sept.-Oct., 1958. "Staphylococcus Sneers at M.D.s Trying to Kill It," *Child-Family Digest*, p. 6.

Wasserman, Michelle. July 30, 1974. "Birth at Home: Medical Politics," *The Boston Phoenix*, pp. 10,12

Whipple, Dorothy V., M.D. Oct., 1975. "Breastfeeding in Today's World," *Journal of American Medical Women's Association*, pp. 936-937.

Wik, Manya. Winter 1973-1974. "Our Home Delivery: An Arctic Adventure," *Expecting*, p. 14.

Windle, William F. Oct. 1969. "Brain Damage by Asphyxia at Birth," *Scientific American*, pp. 77-84.

Wurtman, Richard J. July, 1975. "The Effects of Light on the Human Body," *Scientific American*, pp. 69-77.

Yoho, Bob. Mar. 2, 1974. "Homebirth," *Hutchinson News*, (KS).

Yuncker, Barbara. August, 1975. "Delivery Procedures that Endanger a Baby's Life," *Good Housekeeping*, p. 56.

ABOUT THE AUTHOR

Marilyn A. Moran was born on April 11, 1928 and took her last breath on June 13, 1998. After the birth of her youngest son Patrick, almost 50 years ago, she became the first advocate for husband and wife, do-it-yourself homebirth.

Marilyn introduced the concept of husband and wife do-it-yourself homebirth in this classic, groundbreaking book. She is the author of *Pleasurable Husband/Wife Childbirth: The Real Consummation of Married Love* and *Happy Birth Days: Personal Accounts of Birth at Home the Intimate Husband/Wife Way*.She is the mother of ten children, nine of whom are still living.

Her first seven births were medicated 'deliveries.' Then, in 1967, she had her first Lamaze baby (with no medication) and three years later she had another, this time with her husband in the delivery room. Those two unmedicated births were such a discovery as to the sensations and emotions of birth that she made up her mind never again to give birth in the hospital. Reflecting upon those two births she came to the conclusion that birth is a sexual experience and should rightly take place in the dimly-lit seclusion of the couple's bedroom.

In 1972 that is where her youngest child was born. (She was 44 years old at the time.)

Birth and the Dialogue of Love is a synthesis of the insights and reflections which led up to the author's homebirth and the research she has done since that time.

TWO POEMS

Metamorphosis

Eva,
deluded girl.
Know thee not of thy greatness?

The dregs of thy cup are sweet indeed.
Remember, He had said that all was
"very good."
Drink, girl. DRINK!

Ave, Woman!
Discordant "NO!" forever stilled by
up-ending fiat.
God of creation, I give thee greeting.
God of creation, I salute thee.
Ave!

A Star is Born

Tiny terra firma,
Love chariot speeding on your celestial way.
With carefree riders,
obediently accepting the promptings of the
creative force within them.
The ultimate fission event producing the
ultimate fusion event,
Til in the sky a new star is seen
where once cold planet earth had orbited.

Marilyn Moran

Advent 1980

A NOTE OF APPRECIATION

My sincerest thanks go to two homebirth mothers who helped in the preparation of this book. Diane Lehman did some of the typing. Her daughter, Skye, was born at home April 22, 1977.

Frances Frech checked for typographical errors. (Do hope she got all of them!) Her three youngest children were born at home without medical assistance, Brian, in 1959; Russ, in 1963; and Troy, in 1969. (Incidentally, Frances has a daughter who also has had three do-it-yourself homebirths.)

To them, and to Sandy for her beautiful illustrations, and to all my friends for their interest and enthusiasm for this project I say "Thank you!"

CPSIA information can be obtained
at www.ICGtesting.com
Printed in the USA
LVHW050713271222
735977LV00016BA/981